DEVELOPING

POWER

National Strength and Conditioning Association

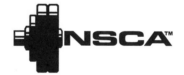

Mike McGuigan

EDITOR

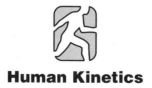

Human Kinetics

Library of Congress Cataloging-in-Publication Data

Names: McGuigan, Mike, 1971- editor. | National Strength and Conditioning
    Association (U.S.), author.
Title: Developing power / Michael McGuigan, Editor.
Description: Champaign, IL : Human Kinetics, 2017. | Series: Sport
    performance series | "National Strength and Conditioning Association." |
    Includes bibliographical references and index.
Identifiers: LCCN 2017019972 (print) | LCCN 2016051696 (ebook) | ISBN
    9781492551058 (ebook) | ISBN 9780736095266 (print) | ISBN 0736095268
    (print)
Subjects: LCSH: Athletes--Training of. | Physical education and training. |
    Physical fitness--Physiological aspects. | Exercise--Physiological
    aspects. | Muscle strength.
Classification: LCC GV711.5 (print) | LCC GV711.5 D474 2017 (ebook) | DDC
    613.7/11--dc23
LC record available at https://lccn.loc.gov/2017019972

ISBN: 978-0-7360-9526-6 (print)

This publication is written and published to provide accurate and authoritative information relevant to the subject matter presented. It is published and sold with the understanding that the author and publisher are not engaged in rendering legal, medical, or other professional services by reason of their authorship or publication of this work. If medical or other expert assistance is required, the services of a competent professional person should be sought.

The web addresses cited in this text were current as of March 2017, unless otherwise noted.

Acquisitions Editors: Justin Klug and Roger Earle; **Developmental Editor:** Kevin Matz; **Managing Editor:** Ann C. Gindes; **Copyeditor:** Annette Pierce; **Indexer:** Dan Connolly; **Permissions Manager:** Martha Gullo; **Graphic Designer:** Angela Snyder; **Cover Designer:** Keith Blomberg; **Photographer (cover and interior):** Tom Kimmel; **Photographs:** © Human Kinetics; **Visual Production Assistant:** Joyce Brumfield; **Photo Production Manager:** Jason Allen; **Senior Art Manager:** Kelly Hendren; **Illustrations:** © Human Kinetics, unless otherwise noted. **Printer:** Versa Press

We thank the National Strength and Conditioning Association in Colorado Springs, Colorado, for assistance in providing the location for the photo shoot for this book.

Human Kinetics books are available at special discounts for bulk purchase. Special editions or book excerpts can also be created to specification. For details, contact the Special Sales Manager at Human Kinetics.

Printed in the United States of America

10 9 8 7 6 5 4 3 2 1

The paper in this book is certified under a sustainable forestry program.

Human Kinetics
Website: www.HumanKinetics.com
United States: Human Kinetics
P.O. Box 5076
Champaign, IL 61825-5076
800-747-4457
e-mail: info@hkusa.com

Canada: Human Kinetics
475 Devonshire Road Unit 100
Windsor, ON N8Y 2L5
800-465-7301 (in Canada only)
e-mail: info@hkcanada.com

Europe: Human Kinetics
107 Bradford Road
Stanningley
Leeds LS28 6AT, United Kingdom
+44 (0) 113 255 5665
e-mail: hk@hkeurope.com

E5178

For information about Human Kinetics' coverage in other areas of the world, please visit our website: www.HumanKinetics.com

DEVELOPING POWER

Contents

PART II Exercises for Power Development

PART III Sport-Specific Power Development

Introduction

The ability to produce maximal muscular power is important in sport performance. One only needs to look at a player performing a slam dunk in basketball or a rugby player changing direction in a game to realize the importance of power for optimal athletic performance. Maximal muscular power refers to the highest level of power (work/time) that can be achieved during muscular contractions. In the applied setting of sport performance, we can think of maximal power as representing the greatest instantaneous power during a single movement performed to produce maximal velocity at takeoff, release, or impact. This includes movements that make up sprinting, jumping, throwing, changing direction, and striking, so power can be considered a critical aspect of many sports.

This book discusses the latest evidence-based guidelines for the assessment and training of muscular power. Using case studies from a range of areas, along with the relevant research on power assessment and development, it provides practitioners with the latest information on how to assess power. Most important, it discusses and provides examples for using this information to design programming. The first chapter sets the scene by introducing the key concepts and underlying science of muscular power. The correct terminology for describing the components of power are outlined. It also discusses contributors to the biological and mechanical basis of power, including morphological factors, neural factors, and muscle mechanics. The relationship between strength and power is another critical theme in the first chapter and throughout the book.

A variety of tests are available to practitioners to assess power in their athletes. Tests, like training, must be specific so that practitioners know they are assessing qualities that are important for a particular sport. Therefore, practitioners should not implement strength and power tests simply for the sake of testing. It is also important to examine the tests used and to avoid choosing them solely because they have been used previously, or because the equipment and the expertise are available. In addition to having reliable, valid, and sensitive tests, it is vital to understand and recognize why each test is included and why it is appropriate. These concepts form the basis of chapter 2, and they aim to provide the reader with an advanced understanding of the assessment of power.

The connection between assessment and programming is critical when designing training programs to develop power. In other words, how do we use the testing results to determine programming? A key purpose of athlete assessment is to obtain insight into the training needs of the athlete. This is an important theme in the book and requires an in-depth understanding of program design. Chapter 3 explains training principles in relation to power development. The integration of power modalities and the periodization of power are also discussed.

It is not just in sports that power is important. Increasing evidence shows that other populations, such as older adults, also experience significant benefits. In addition, as resistance training becomes a more integral part of training programs for youth athletes, practitioners increasingly need to be aware of the role of power training. Power is also a critical physical attribute for tactical personnel such as the armed forces and police, whose jobs frequently require them to move loads quickly. Strength and conditioning practitioners working with different client populations need to know how to assess and to develop muscular power in their clients effectively. Chapter 4 explains the application of power testing and training for two populations with whom strength and conditioning coaches and exercise scientists are increasingly working: youth athletes and older adults. The benefits of power development are now well recognized for these groups, and practitioners can apply the principles discussed in this chapter across a wide range of populations.

For practitioners to be able to train power well, it is critical that they have a range of effective exercises to use with their athletes. A series of chapters provides a technical breakdown of exercises and teaching progressions that develop power. Chapter 5 covers upper body exercises, chapter 6 lower body exercises, and chapter 7 power exercises for the whole body, including the Olympic weightlifting exercises. Being able to coach and able to perform exercises effectively and safely are important parts of the exercise prescription process. Using a range of methods to develop power and choosing appropriate exercises are critical for strength and conditioning practitioners. Some of these methods were introduced in chapters 3 and 4. Chapter 8 extends these discussions by examining more advanced methods of developing power, such as complex training and the use of variable resistance, in more detail.

An often overlooked aspect of improving muscular power is where it fits into training program design. It is important for practitioners to realize that power is not only developed in isolation, but also needs to be considered as part of the overall training program. We have attempted to discuss power in the context of complete program preparation rather than as an isolated component. For example, it is well known that developing muscular strength forms the basis of optimal power development and, as mentioned previously, this is an important theme throughout the book. The final two chapters provide sample training programs that develop power, both for team sports, such as basketball, rugby union, soccer, American football, volleyball, and baseball (chapter 9), and individual sports, such as track and field, swimming, wrestling, golf, rowing, and winter sports (chapter 10). A key feature of these chapters is that they highlight the link between the assessment of power and how assessment can be used to develop training programs.

The contributors to this book are some of the best practitioners and sport scientists in the field of strength and conditioning. They have been invited to contribute to this book because of their expertise and their extensive practical experience working with high-level athletes. They also have the ability to communicate evidence-based information effectively and to apply the latest research in a practical manner. The overall goal of this book is to provide the practitioner with the most cutting-edge and accurate information on power development for improved sport performance. This book will be a valuable addition to the libraries of strength and conditioning practitioners, coaches, and athletes who are interested in evidence-based power training.

PART I

Essentials of Power Development

CHAPTER 1

Nature of Power

Jeffrey M. McBride,
PhD, CSCS

U nderstanding the nature of power is important for understanding athletic performance. Examining power from its inception at the molecular level provides valuable information when designing an optimal training program. Force production is considered as one dimensional in its translation. However, power appears to be a multifaceted system of force, displacement, velocity, and work. These variables should also be put in the context of the constantly changing system in which we examine this phenomenon in terms of muscle lengths, joint angles, and concentric, eccentric, and stretch-shortening cycle patterns of muscle function. Examining power at a molecular level provides a valuable context in which to develop effective ways to maximize the athletic performance of the body as a whole, specifically within the environment in which we have evolved (exclusive of body mass, gravity, and air resistance).

ENERGY

Availability of an energy source has been considered as the primary constituent of the ability to generate power (15, 80) (figure 1.1a). Research shows that we derive this energy within the body from the hydrolysis (unbinding) of adenosine triphosphate (ATP) in which we use the bond energy between the third phosphate group (γ) and the adjacent phosphates (83). The energy within these bonds has been described as being obtained through the processing of primarily carbohydrate and lipids, which we ingest into the body through our natural food sources, with the original source of energy being the sun (19, 44). Because power is work per unit of time, motions or activities that consist of maximal power appear to involve relatively short time frames (9). It appears that the primary energy sources are those that tend to be the most rapidly available. These sources consist of stored ATP within the muscle and the short-term rapid formation of ATP through the donation of phosphate groups from phosphocreatine, which is stored in the muscle as well (36). The additional sources of ATP may be derived from the anaerobic processing of glucose (carbohydrate) stored within muscle and the liver. Energy for sustained levels of small to moderate power outputs for endurance activities could be derived from either the subsequent processing of the end products of anaerobic glycolysis (pyruvate) or beta-oxidation of fatty acids (lipids) stored through the body in adipocytes and anaerobic respiration (Krebs cycle and electron transport chain) (38, 95).

The process of generating external power appears to begin with muscle force and contraction (77) (figure 1.1*b* and 1.1*c*). This muscle shortening could result in motion of our limbs, which is referred to as internal work and this internal work relative to time is then internal power (figure 1.1*d*) (70). The motion of our limbs could then allow for the generation of external forces (forces applied to the ground or external objects through our arms and legs), which could result in the subsequent movement of our whole body's center of mass (COM). External work is the external force generated times the displacement of our COM and relative to time is external power (figure 1.1*e*) (52). This external power is a possible indicator of performance in power activities (e.g., how fast you can run or how high you can jump) (72). In the case of endurance or activities performed repeatedly, mechanical efficiency (the ratio of energy created per unit of time relative to external power) may be our primary variable of concern (45, 63). The primary component of understanding the process of generating power begins with our ability to generate force.

FORCE

Our ability to generate force from a tissue within our body is quite a miraculous process. Muscle could be considered, in some aspects, to be similar to an electric

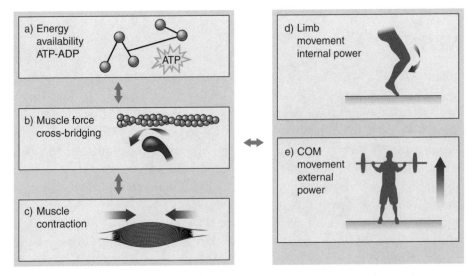

Figure 1.1 *(a)* Energy availability from adenosine triphosphate (ATP), *(b)* force output from actin-myosin cross-bridging, *(c)* muscle contraction, *(d)* limb movement and internal power, and *(e)* whole body center of mass (COM) movement and external power.

motor, but in a molecular form (61). A molecular motor has been reported to take chemical energy (ATP) and use it to perform mechanical work, just as an electric motor uses electricity to perform mechanical work, more specifically, the hydrolysis of ATP, or the removal of the γ-phosphate group, and the subsequent conformational change of myosin (swivel) (11). Within the context of a single cross-bridge, or myosin–actin interaction, the amount of force developed has been reported as approximately 4 pN (7). Thus, in the context of squatting a 100 kg (220 lb) mass, we may be talking about 981 trillion pN or 245 trillion cross-bridges. There appear to be approximately 300 molecules of myosin in each thick filament protein, with each molecule consisting of two heads that attach, swivel, and detach for the production of force (86). It has been reported that these thick filaments are arranged in a pattern to form the smallest repeating functional unit in a muscle, a sarcomere. Some data indicate 2,000-2,500 sarcomeres per 10 mm (0.4 in) of muscle fiber length. While muscles have quite a variation in length, this provides a general construct of the massive number of cross-bridges per fiber, per motor unit, and ultimately, per muscle (94).

The regulatory mechanisms for force output may be vital in determining the amount of work performed per cross-bridge and in what time frame this occurs. Various combinations of mechanisms are reported to determine the power output of a whole muscle. The regulatory mechanisms appear to begin with the nervous system and the action potentials, the electrical signals sent to the muscles (69). Skeletal muscles are typically broken into motor units, that is a motor neuron and all the muscle fibers it innervates. The control of firing rates, the number of action potentials per second, also referred to as rate coding, may be an essential compo-nent in determining peak force and, more important for power, or the rate of force development (RFD) (27, 84). Higher firing rates appear to result in increased rates of force through the summation of muscle twitch force, which typically occurs as the result of a single action potential (27). Thus, the rate at which these muscle twitches occur with respect to each other may determine their summative pattern of peak force and RFD (24).

Studies indicate that inherent capabilities within humans generate action potentials in control of force production, which can be modified by training (91). However, beyond the scope of rate coding, several possible subsequent processes also determine what the peak force and RFD for a muscle may be. The other areas of regulation may include the neuromuscular junction or gap, which appears to consist of neurotransmitter release and generation of action potentials along the membrane of the muscle fibers themselves (26) (figure 1.2). Studies show that within the muscle fiber, the release and sequestering of calcium from the sarcoplasmic reticulum, which is both rate controlled and a trainable phenomenon, may be rate limiting (49). Finally, we may still have a limiting factor in terms of cross-bridge kinetics (67). This may be prescribed by the rate-limiting steps of ATP hydrolysis, the myosin conformational changes, and the detachment–reattachment rates of the myosin head to actin. Thus, a multitude of considerations exist for how force

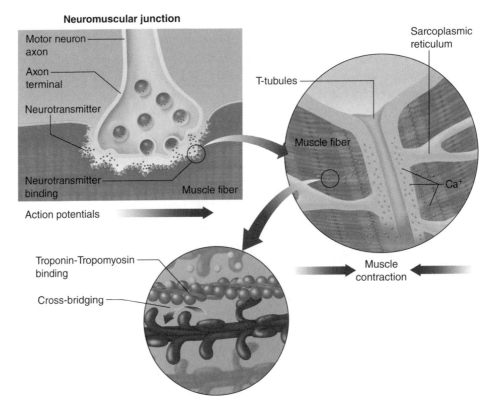

Figure 1.2 Process of muscle contraction from the axon terminal to the neurotransmitter release at the neuromuscular junction to the sarcoplasmic reticulum release of calcium, actin-myosin cross-bridging, and muscle contraction as previously reported.

is created within the neuromuscular system, and subsequently, how work is performed. We should place this force in the context of the actual displacement that occurs within the sarcomere, the muscle fiber, and the whole muscle.

DISPLACEMENT AND VELOCITY

Understanding the various aspects of displacement of the internal system (cross-bridges, sarcomeres, muscle fibers, whole muscle), their translation into the more external aspects of displacement and the velocity of the body's limbs, and then of external objects or the whole body (figure 1.1c, 1.1d, and 1.1e) is important to understanding power. Beginning from an internal perspective, the conformational change in myosin may result in a lever-type system of rotation around a fixed point through an angle of approximately 70 degrees (14). Thus, this has been referred to as the working stroke, force, and displacement (82). The amount of actual displacement for a single cross-bridge interaction has been reported as approximately 5.3 nm (53). Within the context of a single muscle contraction, millions of cross-bridge interactions translate into length changes within sarcomeres, and subsequently, the whole muscle. A sarcomere has been reported as the smallest functional unit within skeletal muscle and often the starting point for the examination of the force–length change relationship that exits in muscle (75). The resting length of a sarcomere has been reported to be 2-3 μm, shortening to 1-1.5 μm and lengthening to 3.5-4 μm. Sarcomeres appear to lie in series and, thus, the shortening of the whole muscle may be a collective of changes in individual sarcomere length. Two possibilities of sarcomere shortening have been reported: One could assume that all sarcomeres shorten the same amount within the context of a single muscle contraction (segment-controlled model) or that possibly various sarcomeres shorten different amounts (fixed-end model), resulting in two possible force–length relationships (75). Variation in sarcomere number in series might also influence the shape and scope of the force–length relationship, and possibly, is influenced by the type of training in which one engages (75).Whole-muscle length changes during contraction occur between a range of 10-20 mm (0.4-.8 in) (46).

Force output across the range of muscle-length change does not appear to be a constant (figure 1.3a). The length changes may result in various states of myosin–actin overlap, and thus, different numbers of actual cross-bridges. Force output appears to occur in a hyperbolic pattern of decreased force output either at very short (ascending limb) or long lengths (descending limb) with maximal force production possibly occurring at some optimal length between these two points (plateau region) (75). There may be an active force production component of a muscle caused by cross-bridge interactions but also passive force production, particularly during lengthening, that could be the result of stretching large structural proteins, such as titin, which appear to connect myosin to the Z-line of the sarcomere (92). This passive force production (or tension) should be a consideration, especially during stretch-shortening cycles within a muscle that commonly occur during athletic movement patterns such running or jumping (23).

To add to the complexity of this condition, a velocity-dependent component may result in force production within a muscle (figure 1.3b). Force output seems to decrease with concentric muscle actions as the velocity of the required shortening increases (4). Thus, a muscle may not be able to produce the same force during an isometric contraction as it can during a high-velocity muscle contraction. However, levels of force production during the concentric phase may exceed this standard pattern during stretch-shortening cycles because of various possible mechanisms initiated during the eccentric phase, such as the stretch-reflex, stored elastic energy (i.e., titin), and cross-bridge potentiation (32).

The eccentric phase of the force–velocity relationship appears to be quite the opposite in that with increasing velocity, force output tends to increase to a certain level and then plateau or decrease during extremely high eccentric velocities (active muscle lengthening) (54). This is because that force might be generated in two distinct ways during concentric vs. eccentric muscle actions. Concentric force production may be caused by cross-bridge swiveling and the attachment–detachment pattern as a result of ATP hydrolysis, as previously discussed. Force

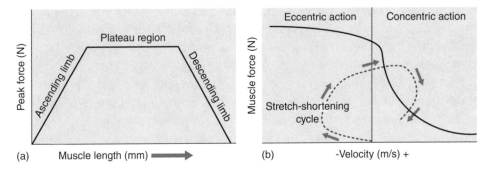

Figure 1.3 *(a)* Muscle force varies as a function of length, increasing (ascending limb), then a plateau region, and then, a subsequent decrease in force (descending limb) in a lengthened position. *(b)* Muscle force during a concentric, an eccentric, and a stretch-shortening cycle muscle action.

production during eccentric muscle actions may occur from forced detachment of the myosin head from actin as a result of tension-induced lengthening of the muscle. This is why eccentric muscle actions have been reported to be associated with muscle damage resulting from forced detachment of myosin heads and the forced lengthening of structural proteins as well (74).

One other factor that may determine the relationship between sarcomere, or muscle fiber, force output relative to velocity of the contraction is the pattern of muscle fiber arrangement relative to the whole muscle–tendon unit (31). Most muscles appear to have a pennated design, in which the muscle fibers are at an angle to the tendon line of the origin and insertion points of the whole muscle (pennation angle). This phenomenon may serve two purposes. First, it may allow for an increased cross-sectional area of muscle fibers within a confined space, referred to as the physiological cross-sectional area. Second, pennation also may result in an anatomical gear ratio, which is the ratio between the shortening velocity of the muscle fiber (or displacement) relative to shortening velocity of the whole muscle (or displacement) (6). In a pennate design, the shortening velocity of the whole muscle has been reported to exceed the shortening velocity of the muscle fiber based on the amount of pennation (pennation angle). The anatomical gear ratio for a muscle may be based on changes in pennation angle, depending on the length of whole muscle and the amount of tension within the muscle. The primary benefit of this variable anatomical gear ratio might be that it extends the range of shortening velocity (at the higher velocities) at which the muscle can produce significant levels of force (13). Both the physiological cross-sectional area and the anatomical gear ratio might be independently influenced by the type of training that an athlete performs (1).

Ultimately, the process of whole-muscle shortening appears to result in joint movement based on the orientation of the origin and the insertion point of the tendons of the muscle (43). The origin and insertion points may also play a role in the amount of angular displacement and the velocity of the corresponding limb (8).

Joint torque (angular effect of force) appears to be a product of the whole-muscle level of force and its corresponding moment arm. Moment arms are defined by the length of a straight line identified from the axis of rotation to a point perpendicular to the line of action (artificial extension of the force vector from the respective whole-muscle contraction). Moment arm lengths seem to be influenced by both the origin and the insertion point of a particular muscle, and the joint angle at which a specific activity takes place (2). Different muscles within the body have various origin and insertion points, most likely based on their required function within the context of a specific joint. Pros and cons may be associated with more distal or more proximal origin and insertion locations (75). For example, a more distal origin or insertion might result in greater torque production, but through a more limited range of joint motion. More proximal locations may result in less torque, but a broader spectrum of torque production across larger joint angles. The other aspect of a distal location is that the velocity of the whole-muscle contraction might need to be higher to result in a higher velocity of movement of the most distal portion of the limb, such as the hand or foot (75). A more proximal location might result in the opposite condition. Thus, this could possibly influence the velocity of the limb in terms of its interaction with external objects such as a ball or the ground itself and also the amount of force applied to these objects (3, 81). This might be the most important aspect of the concepts of displacement and velocity as they apply to the COM displacement and velocity of the whole body.

This, in essence, is considered athletic performance, meaning the displacement or velocity of the body in a vertical and horizontal direction (i.e., jumping and running). The vertical displacement of the COM of the whole body, for example, represents an athlete's jump height, and the horizontal velocity of the COM of the whole body represents running velocity (30, 40). Athletic performances might be derived from the internal displacement and velocity capabilities of cross-bridges, sarcomeres, muscle fibers, whole muscle, joint movements, and then our external values of concern relating to displacement and velocity of the COM of the whole body (40). The external levels of force production, most often referred to as ground reaction forces (GRF), may determine the characteristics of the displacement and velocity of the COM of the whole body. Thus, force, displacement, and time could be combined to determine power output. However, before referring directly to power, we must put the force and displacement in the context of work (force × displacement).

WORK AND TIME

As mentioned previously, the goal of a molecular motor is to convert chemical energy to perform mechanical work (force production and displacement) (29). This is the working stroke. Force production may be a product of cross-bridge interaction and the subsequent sliding (or displacement) of actin, resulting in sarcomere shortening followed by muscle fiber shortening, and finally, whole-muscle shortening, and thus, mechanical work (10). The myosin–actin interaction has been reported to result in approximately 20-50 kJ/mol of free energy, which is assumed to be translated into usable work (working stroke) (51). An important aspect of using free energy derived from cross-bridge interactions may be the ratio between this free energy and the subsequent amount of mechanical work that is actually performed (29, 51). This has been described as the mechanical efficiency of the system. We also may derive free energy from a cross-bridge interaction as a result of the hydrolysis of ATP. ATP, as mentioned previously, is formed within the body through mechanisms of processing primarily carbohydrate and lipids. Energy production (ATP) might be, to a certain extent, determined by changes in lactate concentration (pyruvate generated from anaerobic glycolysis) and also the amount of oxygen transported into the body (aerobic respiration, Krebs cycle, electron transport chain) (28, 55). Lactate can be measured from the blood, and oxygen consumption can be measured by monitoring the amount that enters the body (VO_2) (65). A method for estimating energy expenditure (ATP) is to measure inspired oxygen amounts and express this as a certain level of energy expenditure as 20,202 J/L of oxygen (28). Blood lactate levels used as an estimate of energy expenditure are 60 J × body mass × Δ blood lactate (79).

The other aspect of calculating mechanical efficiency is the mechanical work performed. Calculating work at the muscle level for an athlete may not be possible with current technology. In vitro models of preparations of a single muscle fiber or whole muscle have been used to calculate work (90). However, at a higher level of function, some investigations have determined, or labeled, internal work as the summation of individual body segmental movements as a reflection of the process of whole-muscle contractions around their respective joints (76) (figure 1.4). This process involves assumptions, and the processing occurs through a series of analyses that track body-segmental movements through videography and GRF measurements. Energy changes, and thus internal work, is a measure of the collective changes in potential and kinetic energies of the components of the system (body segments) (93). Another form of assessment is external work (5, 16, 17, 87). This is the summation of the changes in potential and kinetic energies of the COM of the whole body. For the purposes of assessing mechanical efficiency in terms of athletic performance, the measure of external work might be the most practical and the most relevant to athletic performance. Thus, the most meaningful aspect of athletic performance may be the ratio between energy expenditure (lactate and VO_2) and external work. This ratio has been reported in the literature and may be a trainable phenomenon that has an impact on athletic performance (55, 56, 65), especially as it relates to the capabilities to produce work relative to time (power) for endurance-related activities (47). Calculation of external work may also have the most significance for athletic performance in terms of understanding the importance of power (52). Many studies have examined the relationship between power and performance (see chapter 2). What these studies appear to refer to is work performed by the COM of the whole body relative to time. These measures

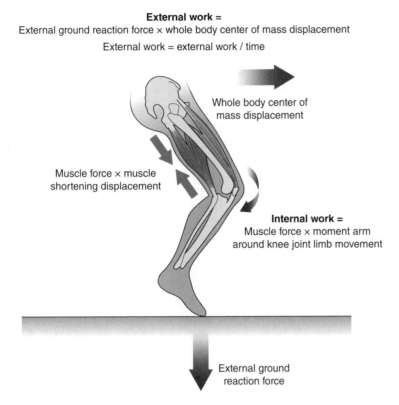

External work =
External ground reaction force × whole body center of mass displacement

External work = external work / time

Whole body center of mass displacement

Muscle force × muscle shortening displacement

Internal work =
Muscle force × moment arm around knee joint limb movement

External ground reaction force

Figure 1.4 Muscle force and shortening, internal work, external work, and external power.

have been calculated from GRFs (force plate measurements) during jumping and running (33, 50). Thus, an athlete's ability to alter kinetic and potential energies (work) could be important in understanding how to improve these variables with respect to time, resulting in increased power (59).

POWER

Power is defined as the rate of performing work and is a product of force and displacement. Another way to think about power is as the amount of force produced during an activity at a given velocity. It was previously mentioned that a myosin–actin interaction (cross-bridge) has been referred to as the *working stroke*. Another common term, and maybe more relevant, is the *power stroke* (34). Power is the culmination of all of the previously covered variables: force, displacement, and time. These three variables may be the essence of what defines athletic performance, and thus, why it has been extensively researched and discussed by both scientists and practitioners (37, 57, 58). Ballistic or semiballistic movement patterns, such as the jump squat and the power clean, have been reported to result in higher power outputs in comparison to heavy-weight (higher % of 1RM) squats (22, 39, 64). Although heavy squats appear to involve relatively high force, the velocity of the movement appears to be lower than the jump squat or the power clean. This lower velocity possibly results in lower values of power (22, 64).

Activities done at a very high velocity also appear to result in lower power levels because that force would be low according to our previous discussion of the force-velocity relationship in the muscle. However, a condition of very high velocity (enough to severely limit power) is not a naturally occurring condition in human movement, unless performed in zero-gravity or microgravity environments (18). It has been reported that running and jumping within the earth's environment results in relatively high power outputs because we must move our whole body in order to run or jump against the gravitational force of the planet (our body weight) (18, 66, 78). This means that a condition of moderate levels of velocity and force may occur simultaneously, as reflected in data from the jump squat using body mass, for example (22, 48). This is an interesting concept initially presented by a study involving jumping in simulated zero-gravity or microgravity environments (18). If you perform a maximal squat, power output appears to be low (high force, low velocity). If you jump or run on the earth, your power appears to be high (moderate force, moderate velocity), but if you jump on the moon, your power appears to be low (low force, high velocity). This hyperbolic relationship may assist in establishing concepts of where and why power occurs in human movement and how to train in order to maximize athletic performance.

Importance of Power

Power may be the essential quality for running fast and jumping high. An organism's ability to generate power might be a product of its evolution in the context of the environment in which it evolves (gravity, atmospheric pressure, and so on) (18, 66, 78). For the purposes of humans, this might be the evolution of the body in the context of the earth's gravitational field. It appears that if athletes want to jump high or run fast, they must generate maximal force through a maximal displacement in a short period of time (39, 78). In addition, they must do this by moving their own body mass against gravity. One's body mass is a force that must be overcome to generate power. Thus, a cross-bridge, a muscle fiber, a whole muscle, a joint movement, and a GRF may be optimized in the context of this environmental arrangement (12, 41, 42, 67).

It is interesting that the concept of maximal force, velocity, and power production might be observed from the level of an individual muscle fiber, to a whole-muscle, to a joint, and finally to the whole body itself (67, 73). Power output capability might be a product of the maximal force a system can produce. As mentioned previously, this could even be brought back to the molecular motor itself. Hydrolysis of ATP has been reported to result in free energy, and thus, mechanical work, all in the context of a certain period of time. However, one must remember that the production of force, whether it be in a single cross-bridge or a whole muscle, must be placed in the context of what the maximal force production capability of the system is, especially regarding velocity. This is because power is a product of force and velocity, and thus, the optimal intersection between these two variables might provide us with our understanding of both where power occurs and how it can be optimized (60, 73).

Maximal Power

An examination of a single muscle fiber indicates that maximal power exhibited may occur at 15%-30% of its maximal force capabilities (35). This also might translate to the whole muscle (42, 68). Even more amazing is that this might translate into the force output of the whole body (41, 68). If an athlete weighs 841 N (85.8 kg [189 lb]) and he or she can generate 1647 N (167.9 kg [370 lb]) of maximal force with the legs in a vertical direction, then the external load at which the athlete can create the most power vertically (jump squat) appears to be 33.8% of this total value ([841 N + 1647 N] × 33.8% = 840.9 N). The answer to this equation is 840.9 N, which is approximately the weight of the athlete and 33.8% of the total value (2,488 N), which is similar to the values of 15%-30% of maximal force production reported in studies of single muscle fibers (35, 71). This means it appears that athletes can generate the most power when they are moving a load approximately equal to their own body weight (18, 20, 22, 25, 62, 64) (figure 1.5). It appears that when the load the athlete trains with increases (1.0-1.5 × BW), peak force increases with coincidental decreases in peak velocity and peak power (64). This is why ballistic power training (e.g., jump squat) might be characterized by training with lower resistances (high peak power) and strength training may be characterized by training with higher resistances (high peak force) (85). This relationship appears to be slightly altered when using the squat (nonballistic) or power clean (semiballistic) as a modality for power training (22, 85), in that the loading is heavier and expressed as a percentage of how much weight the athlete lifts (bar weight or one repetition maximum [1RM]). In the case of the squat, it might be 56% of 1RM, and in the power clean it might be 80% of 1RM (22, 64, 85). Sometimes, the expressions of load are different between the jump squat and the squat or the power clean. The loading for the jump squat, as discussed earlier, is in the context of using the athlete's body weight (BW) as the load (1.0 × BW) or the athlete's body plus some level of additional external loading (1.5 × BW). The loading for the squat or the power clean typically has been placed in the context of how much load is on the bar that the athlete lifts (1RM). In figure 1.5, a load of 1.0 × BW would be equal to 0% of 1RM, or no external load. A load of 1.5 × BW would be equal to (if athlete's mass is 81 kg and has a squat 1RM of 138 kg, for example) of 90% of 1RM (1.5 × 81 kg = 122 kg, 122 kg ÷ 138 kg = 0.90). One can see that in the jump squat, a much lower intensity (load) might be used (0% of 1RM), and in the squat (56% of 1RM) and the power clean (80% of 1RM), a much higher intensity (load) might be used to attain peak power output (22, 85).

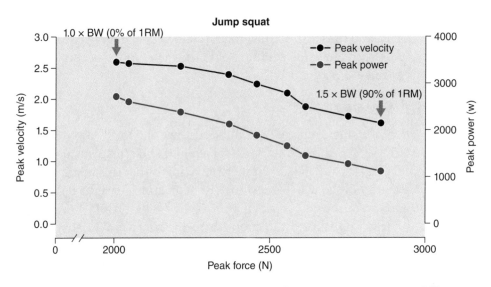

Figure 1.5 Peak force, velocity, and power performing jump squats at different loads from 1.0 × BW (0% of 1RM) to 1.5 × BW (90% of 1RM).

CONCLUSION

When jumping and running, athletes must move their own body weight. Because jumping, running, and most other field-based activities seem to be ballistic in nature, the concepts identified by research using a jump squat model, in terms of force, velocity and power, seem plausible. Therefore, when an athlete jumps or runs with their own body weight, it could possibly be considered power training (i.e. 1.0 × BW or 0% of 1RM). Performing squats or power cleans could supplement jumping and running to develop power, possibly using higher loads as previously mentioned (56% of 1RM or 80% of 1RM respectively).

Research has indicated that training with a load that maximizes power may result in the most significant improvements in power (89); thus, using appropriate loading for each exercise might be an important consideration for programming. Furthermore, it appears that in general, training with multiple loads may be ideal for improving muscle power and velocity across the whole force-velocity spectrum (21, 88). Power may be the essence in which we maximize athletic performance. The information covered in this chapter from a molecular level to the context of jumping and running provides some evidence to support such claims. We take our body and run, jump, swim, ride and climb. This is the nature of power.

CHAPTER 2

Assessment of Power

Sophia Nimphius,
PhD, CSCS,*D

Power has become one of the most commonly discussed aspects of human performance within the strength and conditioning literature. However, measuring power and the colloquial use of the term *power* have been criticized for being misused or wrongly interpreted (22, 36). One should understand the true definition and appropriate context for using the term *power* before assessing power (see chapter 1). In the strength and conditioning literature, power has been measured through a variety of modes (e.g., isokinetic, isoinertial, and ballistic), using various loads, and during a variety of exercises (10, 24). All of these tests and measurements were typically performed in an effort to describe human muscular performance. However, one should always note that the traditional methods of measuring power output have often occurred during repeated maximal efforts over a distance or for a certain amount of time as with a stair-climbing test or Wingate power test (31).

More recently, the strength and conditioning community has begun measuring power output during ballistic exercises, commonly defined as throwing and jumping activities that allow the athlete to accelerate either the bar or the body through the entire range of motion (1, 24). Ballistic exercises themselves are not power activities exclusively, but instead tend to be activities in which we expect external mechanical power or system power to be of a higher value than in other activities that occur at lower velocities. The most common variable that is being measured during these ballistic exercises is net power of the system that has been shown to be a representation of the summed coordinated effort of the individual joint powers (25, 32). Such a measurement has practical advantages (e.g., time, equipment, cost) over direct assessment of individual joint powers.

It is important to understand that power is a measurement and the equivalent of typical measures of athletic performance (e.g., sprint time or vertical jump height). For example, the use of power as a measure of performance in jumping is ill-advised (22) because the explained variance between system power and performance, in this case, jump height, is not large in either male or female athletes (27, 29). However, two individuals with the same jump height (performance) but different magnitudes of power provide additional information about the process of the jump performance. This chapter outlines the factors that are critical to understand when measuring system power within the context of strength and conditioning. The chapter outlines the definition of power, calculation of power, validity and reliability, common direct (lab-based) and indirect (field-based) assessments of power, and examples of data interpretation from data collected during common ballistic assessments.

DEFINING THE TERM *POWER* IN STRENGTH AND CONDITIONING

The colloquial use of the term *power* as a generic trait is commonly misunderstood and interpreted (22, 36). Power is, by definition, the rate of doing work. The unit of measure for work is the joule and the unit of measure for power is the watt (W), defined as a joule per second. Coaches often indicate that athletes are powerful by describing their movements as occurring at a high velocity *relative* to the force they must produce or load they must overcome during the movement. Therefore, movements that occur at slower velocities because of external loads that must be moved (e.g., another person during a tackle or a weighted jump squat) may still be described as powerful because the velocity is high relative to the force required or mass being accelerated. The colloquial use of the term *powerful* was likely a loose interpretation of the mathematical definitions of power. The following mathematical equations associated with power and work can be arranged several ways to derive the various equations for power.

$$Power\ (W) = \frac{work\ (J)}{time\ (s)}$$

Because work is a product of force and displacement, substitution leads to the following equation:

$$Power\ (W) = \frac{force\ (N) \times displacement\ (m)}{time\ (s)}$$

Simplified further (because velocity = displacement ÷ time), we can once again rearrange the equation to what is commonly used or expressed by strength and conditioning practitioners as the equation for power:

$$Power\ (W) = force\ (N) \times velocity\ (m/s)$$

Further, power can be expressed as the mean over the time of the movement, termed mean system power (P_{mean}), or as the highest peak instantaneous system power (P_{peak}). As such, the P_{mean} will always be a lower value and represents the power across the entire movement, whereas the P_{peak} is the power during the highest discrete time point (figure 2.1). For example the P_{mean} during a countermovement has been reported as 765 W, while P_{peak} was reported as 5,014 W (4).

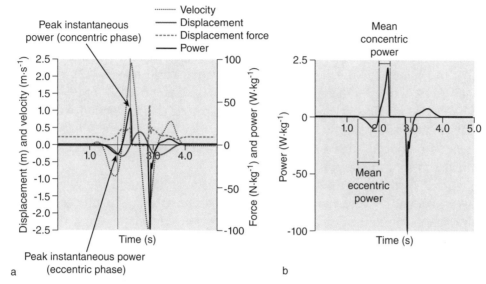

Figure 2.1 A representative countermovement jump with a graphical representation that coincides with standing, lowering during the countermovement, and then extension before takeoff. *(a)* Displacement, velocity, force, and power versus time with the peak power during both the eccentric and concentric phases of the jump are labeled. Notice that the time at which peak power occurs is not the same time that peak velocity and peak force occur. *(b)* Power versus time with an indication of what comprises the entire eccentric and concentric phases. The start and finish of each phase is described in full in text.

The current trend in strength and conditioning training to measure and report P_{mean} or P_{peak} has led to the development of ballistic assessments (e.g., bench press throw and jump) (24). During ballistic assessments, power is often calculated to understand the force–velocity profile of an athlete. However, one should understand that ballistic assessments should not be considered the measurement of power. Instead, one may measure P_{mean} or P_{peak} during these ballistic activities. In fact, system power could technically be measured during any activity except for those that are isometric, where velocity is zero and therefore power is zero. Further, when measuring power, it is critical to fully describe the methods of measurement (discussed in the next section) so the results can be interpreted within the correct context. Other variables, such as force and velocity, should also be presented because power is the mechanical construct of force and velocity (23). Therefore, to correctly interpret power as a measured variable, one must understand the combination of force and velocity changes that elicit the measured power output (see chapter 1 and subsequent section on advantages and drawbacks of power assessment).

MEASUREMENT OF POWER

Much of the strength and conditioning research measuring system power has focused on the P_{peak} and P_{mean} produced during a variety of discrete movements (e.g., squat, jump squat, bench press throw) (22) instead of continuous movements such as cycling or rowing, where power output is measured over repeated efforts. A criticism of using and calculating power only during these discrete movements is that the value does not explain or predict actual performance (22). However, what may be of interest to many practitioners is the change in P_{peak} or P_{mean}, which can reflect adaptations to training when interpreted in conjunction with other variables, such as force or velocity or performance variables such as jump height. The curve produced during a common ballistic movement, a countermovement jump, is shown in figure 2.1.

Figure 2.1 provides the information needed to understand the relationship between commonly measured variables (displacement, velocity, and force) and their relationship to the derived variable of power. To understand how the figure relates to aspects of the jump, consider the displacement curve (figure 2.1) and imagine this curve represents an athlete standing, lowering, jumping to maximum height, landing (then absorbing), and returning to standing height. With this understanding of the phases of the jump relative to the displacement curve, it will be easier to consider the eccentric versus concentric jump phase with respect to power, or any other variable. Further, this particular athlete has two peaks of the force curve (figure 2.1) before take-off. The first peak represents the force exerted to brake the lowering of the body during the countermovement, while the second peak represents the maximal dynamic strength where the athlete summates the forces of the hip, knee, and ankle during the concentric phase of the jump. Such an understanding can be applied to loaded ballistic jumps as well as bench press throws that include a countermovement.

Eccentric and Concentric Phase

The phases of the jump are often described as the portion of the jump with negative change of displacement or positive change of displacement (6). The eccentric phase of the jump (countermovement) has a negative P_{peak} and P_{mean} and commences when the force begins to decrease (figure 2.1). It ends when velocity goes from negative to positive (crosses zero). Simultaneously, this indicates the start of the concentric phase that subsequently ends at takeoff or when force is zero (19).

To derive the power curve shown in figure 2.1, one multiplies the force and velocity data for each sample. The power curve has been isolated in figure 2.1b, where the portions of the power curve that are used to calculate the mean concentric and mean eccentric power values are labeled. The actual calculation of power is relatively simple when velocity and force are directly measured; however, as will be discussed, many methods of measurement can be used to derive the power curve, each with its own advantages and disadvantages.

VALIDITY AND RELIABILITY

Validity and reliability are concepts not only critical to testing in general, but also important in understanding the measurement of system power. Power produced during a variety of physical performance tests have been reviewed extensively in the literature from a validity and reliability perspective (5, 13, 17, 24, 33). Validity can be described as how well a test actually measures the criterion of performance it is intended to measure, while reliability can be described as the ability to reproduce results repeatedly or the consistency of the measure (17). Before the assessment of validity, a measure must be reliable to be worth confirming the validity. All measures of power presented in this chapter are considered to have acceptable reliability. However, with respect to validity, the power measures that are considered in this chapter are split into direct (more valid) and indirect (less valid) measures of system power. When attempting to obtain a valid and reliable measurement of power, even when using direct measures of power, all methodologies are not equal, and the chosen method can still affect the validity and reliability of the measure.

Variables that should be controlled or held constant to increase the reliability of testing include

▶ the testing equipment and the method of calculation,
▶ the instruction to the athlete,
▶ the time of day,
▶ the athlete's fatigue status and familiarity with the testing protocol,
▶ the athlete's experience or training status,
▶ the temperature of testing environment,
▶ the warm-up protocol before testing, and
▶ the order of testing (if other tests are also being performed).

The more controlled the testing environment, the higher the reliability of the testing, which influences the smallest worthwhile change required before determining an improvement in performance. In other words, increasing the reliability of the measure improves the precision, allowing a practitioner to identify smaller changes in athlete performance. Statistically, the smallest worthwhile change can be calculated by multiplying 0.2 times the standard deviation for that performance variable (16). In practical terms, this represents the smallest magnitude change that would have to occur before the change could be considered meaningful (16).

DIRECT AND INDIRECT POWER MEASUREMENT

More focus has been placed on the assessment of power during ballistic activities in strength and conditioning research and practice; therefore, the following description of power assessment will focus on assessment during ballistic activities. However, it is acknowledged that mechanical power output is often measured using a variety of other tests, such as those performed on a cycle ergometer (e.g., Wingate test). Additionally, power has been measured during performance of the Olympic lifts and their derivatives, but because of the unique nature of these exercises and the separate interaction of the bar and the center of mass (COM) of the lifter, special considerations are required when measuring or calculating power during these exercises (18, 20). System power output during ballistic activities is often measured using two broad types of assessment: direct and indirect. From a practical perspective, the decreased cost and increased availability of force plates and linear position transducers (LPT) has led to an increase in practitioners measuring and reporting system power output across a wide variety of tasks using direct measurement.

For an indirect assessment of power, several equations have been derived to predict power output during jumping (table 2.1). However, it is recommended that jump height be used as the performance variable rather than reporting power output using predictive equations. This is because predicted power has greater error and therefore requires a larger smallest worthwhile change to state with certainty that two athletes produced different magnitudes of power (33). For reference purposes,

Table 2.1. Common Equations and Methodologies Used for Predicting System Power Output During Jumping

Name (reference)	Methodology considerations	Formula
Bosco formula (2)	■ Repeated jumps during a given time (15-60s). ■ Test is performed on a contact mat and countermovement depth should be controlled (~90° of flexion), which can be difficult. ■ Hands should be kept on hips.	$Mean\ Power\ (W) = \dfrac{\text{Flight time} \times \text{test duration} \times g^2}{4 \times \text{number of jumps} \times (\text{test duration} - \text{total flight time})}$ where flight time = summation of flight time of all jumps.
Harman formula (15)	■ Single jump for maximal height. ■ Originally developed for squat jump; can use countermovement jump, but this may increase inaccuracy.	$Peak\ Power\ (W) = (61.9 \times \text{jump height (cm)}) + (36.0 \times \text{body mass (kg)}) + 1822$ $Mean\ Power\ (W) = 21.2 \times \text{jump height (cm)} + 23.0 \times \text{body mass (kg)} + 1393$
Sayers formula (30)	■ Single jump for maximal height. ■ May use squat jump or countermovement jump.	$Peak\ Power\ (W) = (60.7 \times \text{jump height (cm)}) + (45.3 \times \text{body mass (kg)}) - 2055$
Lewis formula (12)	■ Single jump for maximal height. ■ Considered least accurate, but widely used.	$Power\ (W) = \sqrt{(4.9 \times \text{body mass (kg)})} \times \sqrt{(\text{jump height (m)})} \times 9.81$

some of the commonly used equations for the prediction of power from a single jump (12, 15, 30) or multiple jumps (2) are listed in table 2.1.

Practitioners should avoid using different activities (modes of movement) or comparison of indirect (Bosco jump test) and direct measures (Wingate cycle ergometer test) of power. For example, the multiple-jump Bosco test results in power outputs different from that measured during a Wingate cycle ergometer tests of the same length on the same participants (15). Recommended best practice is to compare power only within the same type of activity and with the same method of power calculation to ensure valid conclusions. Although the difference in results between the Bosco jump test and Wingate cycle ergometer test for mean power could be explained by differences in stored elastic energy during jumping, one cannot conclude how much of this difference is also a function of comparing direct and indirect measures of power, and it is therefore ill-advised. Because some practitioners will not have access to the equipment required for direct assessments, a comprehensive list of upper body, lower body, total-body, and rotational direct and indirect assessments of power are presented in table 2.2. One should follow a similar recommendation against equating displacement to power for the listed indirect tests of power. Instead, the performance measure reported and used for comparison for an athlete or between athletes should be the jump distance (e.g., broad or long jump) or toss and throw distances.

Table 2.2 Common Methods for Direct and Indirect Assessment of Power

Exercise or test	Purpose	Brief methodology	Variations
UPPER BODY			
Medicine ball chest pass	Upper body explosiveness with indirect (distance) measure of power	Participants sit upright with their backs supported and with legs directly in front or seated on a weight bench with their feet on the floor and their benches inclined at 45°. Mass of medicine ball should be relevant to age or gender (body mass) of participants. Place medicine ball in two hands on chest, and without additional movement, toss the ball for maximal distance (instruct and familiarize participants on angle of toss).	■ Mass of medicine ball ■ Angle of trunk position

(continued)

Table 2.2 *(continued)*

Exercise or test	Purpose	Brief methodology	Variations
UPPER BODY			
Bench press throw	Upper body assessment with direct measure of power*	Participants assume the same positioning as in a bench press while in a Smith machine.* If available, use a magnetic brake to stop the weight after the throw; otherwise, participants should be familiar with both the throw and catch before maximal attempts. Choose between performing a concentric-only throw or allowing a countermovement (similar to that of static or countermovement jump).	▪ Static ▪ Countermovement ▪ Absolute loading profile ▪ Relative loading profile
Upper body Wingate test	Anaerobic capacity with direct measure of power*	Participants sit in a chair facing a cycle ergometer modified for the upper body.* The feet are flat on the floor. Following a warm-up, participants pedal the arm crank to maximal cadence, then add 0.05 kg of load per kg body mass as resistance. Maximal effort will then commence for the required amount of time (typically 30 s).	▪ Length of test
LOWER BODY			
Countermovement jump (CMJ)	Lower body assessment with stretch-shortening cycle with indirect (height)	Participants perform a maximal jump using an arm swing. Measure the maximal reach of a single arm overhead. Then participants jump as high as possible. Participants perform the jump with a self-selected countermovement depth. Subtract the distance between total jump height and reach height to determine jump height.	▪ Single-leg variation

Exercise or test	Purpose	Brief methodology	Variations
LOWER BODY			
Squat (static) jump (SJ)	Lower body assessment without stretch-shortening cycle with indirect (height) measure of power	Participants perform this test same as the CMJ except that they lower to the self-selected depth and hold that position. Upon jumping, they should only move up. If they make a countermovement, negate the trial.	■ Single-leg variation
Broad jump (horizontal jump)	Lower body assessment with stretch-shortening cycle with indirect (distance) measure of power	Participants stand with toes behind a line and then jump forward as far as possible. Participants should use their arms and land under control on both feet. Measure distance from takeoff line to the heel of the closest foot.	■ Repeated jumps or hops ■ Single-leg variations
Countermovement jump (CMJ)	Lower body assessment with stretch-shortening cycle with direct measure of power	Instructions are the same as for the indirect CMJ; however, participants can place their hands either on their hips or on a wooden dowel (or bar where appropriate) so that the power measured is indicative of the lower body. This placement also minimizes variation of results caused by changes in arm swing.	■ Body weight ■ Single-leg variation ■ Absolute loading profile ■ Relative loading profile
Squat (static) jump (SJ)	Lower body assessment without stretch-shortening cycle with direct measure of power*	Instructions are the same as for the indirect SJ; however, participants can place hands either on hips or on a wooden dowel (or bar where appropriate) so that the power measured is indicative of the lower body and minimizes variation of results caused by changes in arm swing.	■ Body weight ■ Single-leg variation ■ Absolute loading profile ■ Relative loading profile

(continued)

23

Table 2.2 *(continued)*

Exercise or test	Purpose	Brief methodology	Variations
LOWER BODY			
Lower body Wingate test	Anaerobic capacity with direct measure of power	Participants perform this on a Monark cycle ergometer.* Bike is adjusted so the leg is just short of full extension at the bottom of the pedal stroke. Following a warm-up, participants pedal to maximal cadence, then add 0.075 kg of load per kg body mass as resistance. Maximal effort then commences for the required amount of time (typically 30 s).	■ Length of test
TOTAL BODY			
Medicine ball toss (overhead or underhand)	Total-body assessment with indirect (distance) measure of power	Numerous methodologies are available that require use of the total body or coordinated movement of the total body to toss or throw a medicine ball for maximal distance. Variations include the standing overhead toss, which is similar to a soccer throw-in or rugby line-out toss or an underhand toss that can be performed either toward the direction of the toss or backward and overhead behind the participant. All variations should be performed with maximal total-body effort.	■ Various release positions ■ Mass of medicine ball
Olympic lifts (snatch, clean and jerk) and derivatives	Total-body assessment (primarily lower-body with direct measure of power*	Measure the hang variations directly as described in table 2.3 and chapter 7. Participants should be proficient in the techniques before performing these exercises.	■ Exercise variations (e.g., hang clean) ■ Absolute loading profile ■ Relative loading profile

Exercise or test	Purpose	Brief methodology	Variations
ROTATIONAL			
Rotational medicine ball toss	Rotational assessment with indirect measure of power	This is commonly performed by athletes in sports with a high rotational component, such as baseball and softball. From a side-on stance, participants toss the ball for maximal distance. Ball should be in both hands and start behind the athlete at a height between waist and shoulders, similar to a batting stance.	■ Mass of medicine ball

Participants should perform these methods only after appropriate familiarization and warm-up in line with suggestions for improvement of reliability of testing. *Direct measures of power use one of the methodologies that directly assess variables to calculate system power as described in table 2.3.

Consistent with the information provided thus far on power measurement, if possible, practitioners should not use the equations in table 2.1 or any indirect (predictive) measure of power exclusively. The direct measurement of system power is considered the most valid measure capable of effectively detecting minimal differences or smallest worthwhile changes in system power following a training block or for comparison between athletes. Considering the types of direct measures used to report power output (5, 8, 24), the reliability and validity of these methodologies should also be considered. An understanding of the advantages and disadvantages of various methodologies for the direct assessment of power is described in table 2.3.

Using the information provided, final recommendations can be made to practitioners to ensure they use valid and reliable system-power measurements to assess athletes. However, not all practitioners will have access to the equipment described; therefore, they should use a combination of the most valid and reliable methods possible while understanding the subsequent limitations.

The following summarizes the overall recommendations for direct measurement of system power during ballistic activities:

▶ Direct measurement of velocity using an LPT, and most accurately two LPTs, to remove error caused by horizontal displacement in conjunction with direct force measurement is best practice when assessing velocity of the bar (5).

▶ A single LPT, either with or without the use of a force plate, can measure the power output of movement that is primarily linear (vertical). Other movements, such as a clean or snatch, that have as much of 10% of the work done horizontally (13), could result in an inflated velocity and power measure if assessed using only a single LPT.

Table 2.3 Advantages and Disadvantages of Various Direct Measures of System or Mechanical Power

Equipment	Advantages	Disadvantages
2 (or 4) LPTs and FP	Direct measure of force and displacement (to calculate velocity). Includes measurement of horizontal displacement (or velocity) during movements that are not fully linear (vertical or horizontal only).	Most expensive setup and requires designated space because of equipment requirements.[a]
1 LPT and FP	Direct measure of both force and displacement (to calculate velocity). Combination is valid assessment of power based on the bar velocity during ballistic movements.	Assumption that movements are fully linear (e.g., not ideal for Olympic variations) and bar velocity is representative of center of mass velocity.[a]
FP only	Highly reliable and valid for both weightlifting (from hang positions) and ballistic movements. Valid assessment of the power based on the center of mass velocity.	Mathematical manipulation (forward dynamics) to calculate power that could result in error associated with underestimation of power.[b]
LPT only (or 2-D kinematic analysis*)	Relatively inexpensive. Reliable measure of velocity if movement is primarily linear (vertical or horizontal only).	Mathematical manipulation (inverse dynamics) can cause magnification of error in calculation and often overestimation of power.[a]
Accelerometer	Relatively inexpensive. Reliable measure of jump height during CMJ.	Reliability and bias of velocity and power measures increase minimal difference required when assessing changes in power.[a]

Linear position transducer (LPT). Force plate (FP). *Two dimensional (2-D) kinematic analysis refers to using a marker on the athlete's hip (greater trochanter) to represent the change in the athlete's center of mass. [a]Measurement of power is based on the velocity of the bar and therefore does not include movements independent of the barbell. [b]Measurement of power is based on the velocity of the center of mass (system) and therefore does not consider barbell movement.

▶ Use caution when using accelerometers to measure system power because of the potentially large errors that may make it difficult to compare between or evaluate changes in power following an intervention (8).

▶ If the system or mechanical power of the center of mass is of greater interest than the mechanical power of the bar, then a methodology that uses only a force plate may be most applicable and may differentiate from power improvement based on changes in bar path (technique) versus changes in the ability to apply force to the ground (18).

▶ Sampling frequency should be above 200 Hz, particularly if only peak values (e.g., peak power, peak velocity) are of interest. Best practice is a sampling frequency at or above 1,000 Hz when you intend to assess rate of force development (24).

▶ The chosen valid and reliable methodology should be identical both within testing sessions and between testing sessions to ensure that results can be compared.

REPORTING POWER RESULTS

When calculating power, the units can be expressed in terms of either an absolute measure (W) or normalized by a factor such as body mass ($W \cdot kg^{-1}$), termed ratio scaling. The use of allometric scaling has been proposed as a way to understand a variable independent of body size and has been a topic of great discussion in the literature (9, 21, 26). Allometric scaling is defined as normalizing data according to dimensionality to remove the effect of body size by normalizing the variable by dividing it by body mass raised to the two-thirds ($BM^{-0.67}$) (26) . However, before using allometric scaling for normalization, consider its advantages and disadvantages. For example, a potential issue with using the proposed exponent ($BM^{-0.67}$) is the known variations in body size, particularly lean muscle mass, across genders or different athlete groups (because of body type) that can affect the ability of the exponent ($BM^{-0.67}$) to correctly remove the effect of body size (26). To handle this potential issue, it is suggested to derive an exponent instead of using the common $BM^{-0.67}$ exponent. However, derived exponents lack generalizability because derived exponents may be specific to the characteristics of the group used to derive them, such as gender, age, body mass index, and training history (9, 37). Practically, this means practitioners may not be able to compare performance data if it normalized using either a proposed or a derived allometric exponent if their athletes' body size characteristics are different. Because data comparison is a common aspect of performance testing, understanding the method of normalization used is critical.

Practitioners should understand both that a bias may exist in ratio scaling (normalizing to body mass) and the potential implications for their larger and smaller athletes if ratio scaling is the chosen normalization method. However, when relating results to predictions of performance, ratio scaling has provided a better relationship between normalized variables and performance than allometrically scaled variables and performance (9). If one needs to eliminate the potential effect of body size to remove confounding factors related to very small or very large athletes, then either a derived or proposed allometric scaling can be considered (9). Before applying allometric scaling, practitioners should meet assumptions, and understand the implications and use of allometric scaling, and read a variety of resources (3, 26, 34).

PRESENTATION OF TESTING DATA

Beyond data normalization, another important consideration with respect to the presentation of power data is the context of the test performed. As previously mentioned, all movements except those without velocity (isometric) have a power output. However, the comparison between modes of exercise or loadings may best be evaluated using a standardized score as commonly used to compare different aspects of physical performance (e.g., speed to endurance). A standardized score, also termed a Z-*score*, calculates how many standard deviations the value is above or below the mean. You can calculate the Z-score using the following equation, where x is the score to be standardized, μ is the mean, and σ is the standard deviation:

$$z - score = \frac{x - \mu}{\sigma}$$

The raw data for an athlete is presented in figure 2.2, and two versions of this athlete's data standardized are shown in figure 2.3. Figure 2.2 shows the power profile, or power output, across a range of loadings during the jump squat (figure 2.2) as commonly assessed in research (11). In addition, these results have been standardized (figure 2.3), allowing a coach to understand how an athlete is improving at each load relative to the team. The difference between figure 2.3a and 2.3b is caused by the means and standard deviations used to calculate the Z-score. The team means and standard deviations at each load during pre-, mid- and post-testing, respectively, were used to calculate the Z-scores in figure 2.3a, while in figure 2.3b only the means and standard deviations at each load during pretesting were used to calculate subsequent Z-scores at pre-, mid-, and posttesting.

The data in figure 2.2 shows a power profile shift upward from pretesting to midtesting and then shifted up further (but not as substantially across all loads) from midtesting to posttesting. In particular, power production in the counter-movement jump (body mass–only load) went up vastly. The two blocks of training between pre- and midtesting were strength-focused blocks, and the two blocks of training from mid- to posttesting were power-focused blocks, explaining the shift in either the whole curve or the higher-velocity, low-load end of the curve (14, 28). A discussion with respect to training the force–velocity curve and the effect on power occurs in chapter 3. This demonstrates how measured power data can be presented to display or determine specific questions about the efficacy of training. Further case studies are provided in chapters 9 and 10.

It is important that practitioners understand the different information that methods of data presentation convey. If the purpose of the testing data is to show the development of an athlete over time, independent of team changes, then either presentation of the raw data as previously described (figure 2.2) or keeping a constant (e.g., pretesting) mean and standard deviation is advised (figure 2.3b). If one is trying to understand how an athlete is developing in comparison to the team over time, then one should use a moving team mean and standard deviation

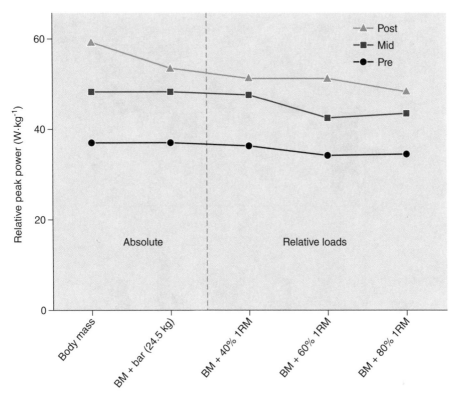

Figure 2.2 Example of a power profile with absolute and relative loads of an athlete at various points in a season (pre-, mid-, and posttesting).

at each time of testing (e.g., pre-, mid-, and posttesting) (figure 2.3*a*). Figure 2.3*a* provides an example of how the mean and standard deviation or the "goal post of comparison" constantly changing can affect our interpretation of the individual athlete's improvement. For example, in figure 2.2, it is clear that at both absolute loads and relative loads, the athlete improved at pre-, mid- and posttesting points. However, when evaluating this athlete relative to the improvements of the team (figure 2.3*a*), this athlete performed below or near the team mean until the final testing when they improved vastly, not only compared to their own scores (as is indicated in figure 2.2) but also in comparison to the team (figure 2.3*a*), as indicated by their high Z-scores at each load. This presentation of data is quite different from that in figure 2.3*b*, which indicates that in comparison to the team mean at pretesting, they far exceeded this baseline level at mid- and post-testing sessions despite starting near the team mean at pretesting.

Figures 2.3*a* and 2.3*b* represent different ways of presenting data, but both are potentially useful for understanding athlete improvement (are they improving more or less than teammates versus more or less than from where the team started?). Understanding the purpose of your testing and the question you want to answer by using that data helps you choose the appropriate data presentation. This concept is

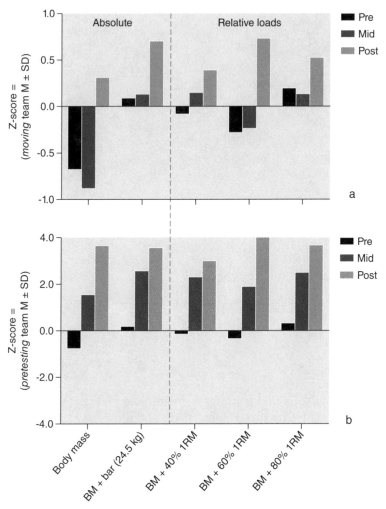

Figure 2.3 Example of standardized scores (Z-score) of an athlete at various absolute and relative loads calculated with either (a) a moving team mean and standard deviation at pre-, mid- and posttesting, or (b) using a static team mean and standard deviation at each load from pretesting.

critical for gathering data that aids rather than detracts from your ability to make decisions on training and athlete improvement. Further, one may compare the normalized power output of an athlete to the ranges that are commonly produced under the same loads or modes of exercise, as discussed in chapter 3.

ADVANTAGES AND DRAWBACKS OF POWER ASSESSMENT

It is common to compare the power output of various ballistic movements and loading paradigms in an effort to understand the power profile of an athlete as previously presented in figure 2.2. These power profiles are regularly used to discuss various loads that maximize power (7, 11, 35). However, the drawback of this approach is a potential overemphasis on finding the load that maximizes power. Instead, a mixed-methods approach to effectively train this proposed power spectrum is recommended (14). In fact, power, being a variable of mechanical construct, is just a description of how the force–velocity profile shifts with various loads or during various activities and is less a determinant of performance. To understand this further, figure 2.4 shows two athletes of similar body mass who produced similar power outputs (within 1%) during a vertical jump but had an approximately 10% difference in performance (jump height). Therefore, only knowing P_{peak} of these athletes would not provide additional insight into how they produce their power or the differences that underpin their performance.

To understand the determinants of their performance, we could look directly at impulse, but this provides the same information as the eventual jump height. However, an aspect of impulse that may provide insight—time—can be evaluated in figure 2.4. Specifically, understanding time with respect to performance can

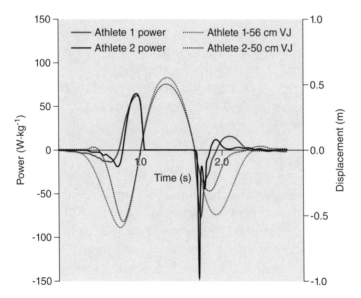

	Peak velocity	Relative peak force	Relative peak power	Force at peak power	Velocity at peak power	Ratio of flight time to contraction time
Athlete 1	2.93	62.63	21.07	21.57	2.90	0.64
Athlete 2	2.75	64.78	21.34	24.29	2.67	0.85
% Difference	6%	-3%	-1%	-12%	9%	-28%

Figure 2.4 Comparison of two athletes with identical power outputs normalized to their body mass. Observe the differences in the displacement and power curves as well as the percentage difference of various chosen variables. This provides an example of how power as a standalone variable can be misleading in the comparison of athletes and should be accompanied with a comprehensive understanding of how the athlete develops his or her power.

be described using a ratio of flight time to contraction time (FT:CT) (4). Although athlete 1 has a higher jump performance, through investigation of other variables we may hypothesize that this athlete may strive to improve rate of force development (RFD) or should be assessed using a shorter stretch-shortening cycle (SSC) activity to see whether he or she still has the capacity to perform when time is restricted or limited, such as with a drop jump. In sport, time limitation is an important consideration with respect to performance. For example, if two people have the same capacity for jump height, but one can jump the same height with less preparation time (or contraction time), that individual may have an advantage in seeing the angle a ball will bounce during a rebound or when diving to save a goal. This is because the individual who can jump with less preparation time can move with the same capacity but in a shorter amount of time. The data that may be used to draw such conclusions can come from both inspection of the displacement–time curve and direct analysis of the FT:CT, which in the previous example demonstrated a 28% difference between these two athletes, while their actual performance (jump height) only differed by 10% (figure 2.4). However, it was inspection of many of the variables that characterize the performance beyond just power that helped to draw such conclusions. Therefore, power has a great capacity to describe the combination of force and velocity into a single simple metric, but deeper analysis is required to understand underlying determinants of athlete performance. For this reason, power, as a variable, should never be used exclusively, and justifies the presentation of results using a force-velocity or evaluation of different metrics beyond that of power.

CONCLUSION

Although power is a highly discussed and measured variable, its usefulness is partially determined by the methodology chosen and partially determined by the intent or question one plans to answer with the measurement of power. Valid and reliable methodologies are used to accurately assess P_{peak} and P_{mean} during a variety of tasks. Practitioners who cannot directly measure power can choose indirect power assessments while understanding their limitations. Further, one must consider the best method to present results to provide meaningful information about the physical characteristics of the athlete. Understanding the limitations of the equipment and methods used to measure power, the best methods to express the data once it is collected, and the underpinning information variables, such as force and velocity, will allow practitioners direct insight into the mechanism by which athletes produce their performance.

CHAPTER 3

Periodization and Power Integration

G. Gregory Haff,
PhD, CSCS,*D,
FNSCA

Periodization is a widely accepted theoretical and practical paradigm for guiding the preparation of athletes (11, 38, 91). Although periodization is both widely accepted and considered an essential tool for guiding training, coaches and sport scientists often misunderstand it and misapply it. While this confusion has many causes, the most important appears to be centered on what periodization is and how it differs from programming and planning (10). Planning is the process of organizing and arranging training structures into phases in order to achieve a targeted goal. Programming is the application of training modes and methods into this structure. Periodization, on the other hand, contains elements of both planning and programming, in that it defines the training structure, the modes, and the methods used within the global training plan. Based on this construct, the manipulation of sets, repetitions, and training loads would be considered programming, not periodization as it is sometimes falsely defined in the literature (24, 25, 59). Periodization is an inclusive theoretical and practical construct that allows for the management of the workloads of all training factors in order to direct adaptation and elevate performance at appropriate times through the integrative and sequential manipulation of programmatic structures (38, 45, 76, 78, 94).

The ability to manipulate training factors in a structured fashion allows periodized training plans to target several distinct goals. These include (i) the optimization of the athlete's performance capacity at predetermined times, or the maintenance of performances across a season, (ii) targeting the development of specific physiological and performance outcomes with precise training interventions, (iii) reducing overtraining potential through the appropriate management of training stressors, and (iv) facilitating long-term athlete development (32-34, 38, 91, 94). The multidimensional application of training interventions in an integrative and sequential manner largely affects the ability of periodized training models to accomplish these goals. While a central component of an appropriately designed periodized training plan is training variation, one should avoid random or excessive variation because this will mute performance gains (94) and lead to an increased risk of injury (77). Training variation should be logical and systematic so that the training responses are modulated while accounting for fatigue and elevating performance at appropriate times (38).

To apply these principles to maximize power development, one must consider several key aspects of periodization, planning, and programming. This chapter discusses the general principles of periodization, the hierarchical structure of periodization cycles, and understanding the periodization process, approaches to planning used in periodization, models of periodization, fundamentals of power development, and planning training and power development.

GENERAL PRINCIPLES OF PERIODIZATION

The ability to develop specific physiological adaptations and translate those adaptations into performance outcomes is largely dictated by the ability to sequence and structure the periodized training plan in order to manage both recovery and adaptive processes (22, 24, 65, 78, 94). Because it is well documented that peak performance can only be maintained for a relatively small period of time (8-14 days) (7, 16, 51, 71-73), the sequential structure of the training plan becomes a critical consideration for periodization (13-15, 78, 94, 106). Ultimately, the average intensity contained in the training plan is inversely related to the magnitude of the performance peak and the duration with which that peak can be maintained (23, 45, 94). Three basic mechanistic theories can be used to understand how periodized training programs can manage the recovery and adaptive processes: the general adaptive syndrome (32-34, 38, 94, 113), the stimulus-fatigue-fitness-adaptation theory (32-34, 38, 89, 94), and the fitness–fatigue paradigm (18, 32-34, 38, 94, 113).

General Adaptive Syndrome (GAS)

One of the foundational theories that underpins the periodization of training is Hans Selye's general adaptive syndrome (GAS) (38, 94, 115). The GAS describes the body's specific responses to stress, either physiological or emotional (89). While the GAS offers a potential model that explains how the body adapts to training stimuli, it does not explain all the responses to stress that occur (figure 3.1) (94).

When applying GAS to training theory, it is important to note that the body appears to respond in a similar fashion regardless of the type of stressor that is applied (38). If you introduce new training stimuli (e.g., stress) to the athlete, the initial response, *or alarm phase*, results in a reduction in the athlete's performance capacity as a result of the accumulation of fatigue, stiffness, soreness, and reductions in available energy stores (38). The *alarm phase* initiates the adaptive processes that lead into the *resistance phase*. If training is programmed correctly, the athlete's

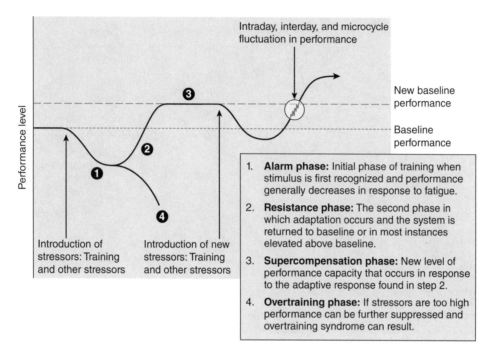

Figure 3.1 The general adaptive syndrome and its application to periodization.

Reprinted, by permission, from G.G. Haff and E.E. Haff, 2012, Training integration and periodization. In NSCA's guide to program design, edited for the National Strength and Conditioning Association by J. Hoffman (Champaign, IL: Human Kinetics), 216. Adapted from Yakovlev (110), Verkishansky (104), Rowbottom (81), and Stone et al. (94).

overall performance capacity will be maintained or elevated (i.e., supercompensate) as a result of being able to adapt to the applied training stimuli. Conversely, if the training stimuli are excessive or randomly applied, the athlete will be unable to adapt to the training stress. Consequently, performance capacity will continue to decline, resulting in a state of *overtraining* (28). An additional consideration is that the athlete's ability to adapt and respond to training stimuli can be affected by other stressors (e.g., interpersonal relationships, nutrition, career pressures) because all stressors are additive.

Stimulus-Fatigue-Recovery-Adaptation Theory

When a training stimulus is applied, a general response occurs, which can be explained by the stimulus-fatigue-fitness-adaptation theory (figure 3.2). Whenever a training stimulus is applied, fatigue ensues, resulting in a reduction in both preparedness and performance. The reduction in both performance and preparedness is proportional to the magnitude and duration of the workload (38). As the recovery process begins and the accumulated fatigue dissipates, both preparedness and performance increase. If, after the recovery process is complete, no new training stimulus is encountered, both preparedness and performance will decline and a state of involution will occur.

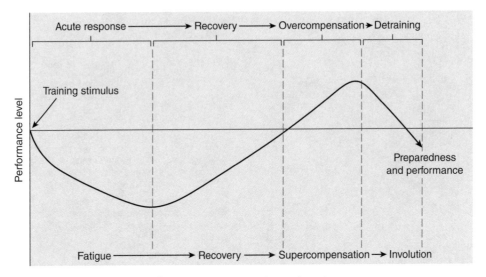

Figure 3.2   The stimulus-fatigue-recovery-adaptation theory.

Reprinted, by permission, from G.G. Haff and E.E. Haff, 2012, Training integration and periodization. In *NSCA's guide to program design,* edited for the National Strength and Conditioning Association by J. Hoffman (Champaign, IL: Human Kinetics), 216. Adapted from Yakovlev (110), Verkishansky (104), Rowbottom (81), and Stone et al. (94).

Careful inspection of the base concept reveals that the magnitude of the training stimulus affects the length of the recovery-adaptation portion of the process (38). For example, a large training load will cause a large amount of fatigue, which will require more recovery time before the recovery-adaptation process can occur (81, 94). Conversely, if the training load is light, the athlete will experience less accumulated fatigue and the recovery-adaptation process will proceed more rapidly. In the training literature, this response is often referred to as a delayed or residual training effect (38, 81, 94). One can modulate delayed training effects by manipulating the training program to ensure that preparedness and performance are supercompensated at key time increments (33). Central to the ability to modulate residual training effects is how one integrates and sequences the workloads in the periodized training program.

While the stimulus-fatigue-recovery-adaptation theory is often considered in a global context, one should remember that this general response pattern occurs as a result of a single exercise, training session, microcycle, mesocycle, and macrocycle (38). Additionally, it is important to note that complete recovery is not required before encountering another training stimulus (74). In fact, it is recommended that coaches modulate training intensities by scheduling heavy and light training days in order to facilitate recovery, maximize adaptive potential (17, 26), and further develop fitness (38). The ability to maximize adaptive responses to training relies on the ability to take advantage of the recovery-adaptation process by manipulating training factors within the programmatic structure that are used in the context of the periodized training plan. This concept is a foundation from which several sequential periodization models presented in the literature have been developed (78, 102-105).

Fatigue–Fitness Paradigm

The interrelationship between fitness, fatigue, and preparedness are partially explained by what Zatsiorsky (113) termed the *fatigue–fitness paradigm*. This paradigm gives a more complete picture of the athlete's response to the training stimulus (18). Central to the understanding of the paradigm are the two aftereffects of fitness and fatigue, which summate to dictate the athlete's overall preparedness (18, 113). Classically, these aftereffects are presented as one fatigue–fitness curve (figure 3.3) (18, 113). However, it is more realistic that multiple independent fitness and fatigue aftereffects occur in response to training and exert a cumulative effect on the preparedness curve (figure 3.4) (18, 38).

The existence of multiple fatigue and fitness aftereffects may partially explain the individual responses to variations in training stimuli (38). Stone, Stone, and Sands (94) suggest that different training targets have different aftereffects, and that targeted training interventions have the ability to modulate which aftereffects occur and how an athlete can progress in preparedness throughout the training plan. These training-induced aftereffects are also referred to as residual training effects, and serve as the foundation for the theories that underpin sequential training (48, 49, 103, 106).

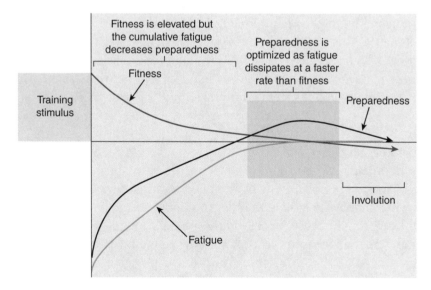

Figure 3.3 The fitness-fatigue paradigm.

Reprinted, by permission, from G.G. Haff and E.E. Haff, 2012, Training integration and periodization. In NSCA's guide to program design, edited for the National Strength and Conditioning Association by J. Hoffman (Champaign, IL: Human Kinetics), 219. Adapted from Stone et al. (94) and Zatsiorsky (115).

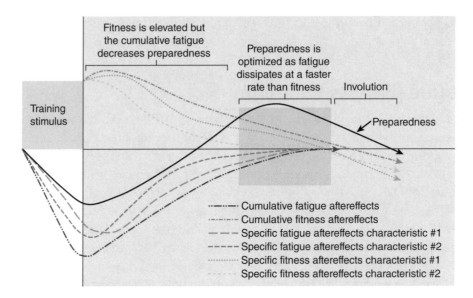

Figure 3.4 Modified fitness–fatigue paradigm depicting multiple training aftereffects.

Reprinted, by permission, from G.G. Haff and E.E. Haff, 2012, Training integration and periodization. In NSCA's guide to program design, edited for the National Strength and Conditioning Association by J. Hoffman (Champaign, IL: Human Kinetics), 219. Adapted from Stone et al. (94) and Zatsiorsky (115).

Sequential training theory suggests that the rate of decay of a residual training effect can be maintained by a minimal training stimulus or through the periodic dosing of the training factor in order to modulate the athlete's preparedness. One can modulate the rate of decay of a given residual training effect by manipulating the training stimulus. In sequential modeling, it appears that residual training effects can be magnified if specific training stimuli are sequenced and integrated correctly, resulting in a delayed training effect or a phase-potentiation effect (38).

When the GAS, stimulus-fatigue-fitness-adaptation theory, and the fitness-fatigue paradigm are used collectively to examine periodization models, it is clear that the modulation of the adaptive responses is accomplished through careful planning. The training plan must be designed to develop various fitness characteristics while managing fatigue in order to maximize the performance capacity of the athlete (38). The ability to control the athlete's level of preparedness centers on the ability to manage training loads in order to modulate both fatigue and fitness aftereffects (78). When designing the training plan, it is essential to consider the training interventions, the actual sequential pattern, and the integration of the training interventions in order to maximize the performance capacity and fitness aftereffects, while minimizing accumulated fatigue.

HIERARCHICAL STRUCTURE OF PERIODIZATION CYCLES

The periodization of training is facilitated by a hierarchical structure that allows for several distinct interrelated levels that can be used in the planning process (table 3.1). Each level of the periodization process should be based on the training goals established for the athlete or team. Conceptually, these levels of organization start with a global context and then progress into smaller more defined structures. Seven hierarchical structures are typically used in the periodization of training.

The highest level of the hierarchical structure is the multiyear plan, which is most typically built around the Olympic quadrennial cycle (11, 52, 74, 76, 83, 113). This cycle presents the athlete's longer-term training goals and uses multiple annual training plans. The next hierarchical level is the annual training plan, which

Table 3.1 Hierarchical Structure of Periodized Training Plans

Level	Name	Duration	Description
1	Multiyear training plan	2-4 years	This plan lays out the long-term goals for the athlete. The most common multiyear plan is the 4-year quadrennial plan.
2	Annual training plan	Several months to a year	This plan outlines the entire year of training. It can contain 1-3 macrocycles depending on the number of competitive seasons contained in the training year. It typically contains preparation, competition, and transition periods.
3	Mesocycle	2-6 weeks	This medium-sized cycle is often referred to as a block of training. The most typical duration for the mesocycle is 4 weeks. Regardless of length, the cycle consists of linked microcycles.
4	Microcycle	Several days to 2 weeks	This smaller training cycle consists of several training days and typically lasts 7 days.
5	Training day	1 day	A training day is designed in the context of the microcycle goals and defines when training sessions are performed within the microcycle.
6	Training session	Minutes to hours	A training session contains all the scheduled training units. It can be performed individually or within a group. If the training session contains >30 min of rest between training units, then multiple session would be performed.
7	Training unit	Several minutes to hours	A training unit is a focused training activity. Warm-up, agility, strength training, and technical drills are examples of training units. Several training units can be strung together to create a training session.

Adapted from Bompa and Haff (11), Haff (34), Haff and Haff (38), Issurin (50), and Stone et al. (94).

contains the training structures within an individual training year (22, 32-34, 38, 76, 81). Annual plans can contain one or more macrocycles, depending on how many competitive seasons are contained in the annual training plan (11, 50). Each macrocycle is then subdivided into three periods: preparation, competition, and transition (32, 38). The preparation period is divided into the general preparation and specific preparation phases. The general preparation phase develops a general physical base and is marked by high volumes of training, lower training intensities, and a large variety of training means (49, 65). The specific preparation phase targets sport-specific motor and technical abilities, which are built on the foundation of the general preparation phase (38). The competition period is structured to slightly improve or maintain the physiological and sport-specific skills established in the preparation period (38). This period is typically subdivided into the precompetition and main competition phases. Conceptually, the precompetition phase is a link between the preparation period and the main competition phase (38). Finally, the transition phase is the most important linking phase and can bridge either multiple macrocycles or annual training plans (11, 74, 81).

The next hierarchical structure, the mesocycle, is sometimes referred to as a medium-duration training cycle (48, 49, 61, 76, 94, 104, 113, 115). It is often referred to as a block of training and is a central training cycle in the block-periodization model (38, 50). Mesocycles typically contain two to six microcycles, which are next in the hierarchy (38). Each microcycle is made up of both training days and sessions, which contain the individual training units. These last components of the hierarchy form the foundation for the whole training system and outline the main training factors delivered (38, 50).

UNDERSTANDING THE PERIODIZATION PROCESS

When we look at the overall periodization process, we must consider it in the context of three basic levels: periodization, planning, and programming (figure 3.5).

The first level is periodization, which dictates the long-term development of the athlete across the multiyear or annual training plan. This level includes the overall breakdown of the preparation, competition, and transition periods. It may also include the travel and testing schedule. The second level is planning, which forms the foundation for choosing the training model used to design the training structures. This can include parallel, sequential, block, or emphasis training models. The third level, programming, contains the basic training structures, such as the modes and methods used. This level contains the training loads (i.e., intensity and volume) as well as the structures (e.g., complexes, cluster sets) and exercises used to construct the training interventions.

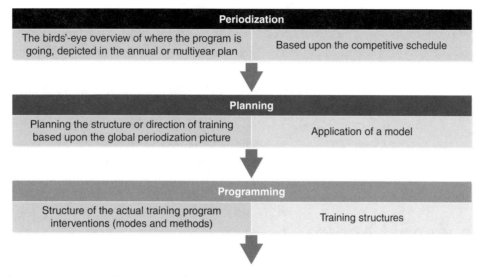

Figure 3.5 Interrelationship of periodization, planning, and programming.

APPROACHES TO PLANNING USED IN PERIODIZATION

When examining the periodization process, and in particular the planning of training, numerous models can be used in accordance with the overall periodized plan. These include parallel, sequential, and emphasis approaches to designing training interventions (10, 53).

Parallel Approach

Coaches use the parallel approach to train multiple biomotor abilities simultaneously and to train all targets across the annual training plan (figure 3.6). Using this approach, all targeted biomotor abilities may be trained within one training session, training day, series of training days, or microcycle. Sometimes this approach is called a concurrent or complex parallel approach (10).

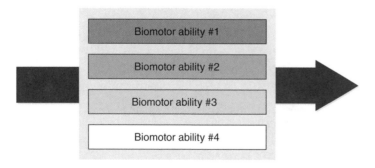

Figure 3.6 Parallel training approach.

One of the issues with the parallel approach is that in order to continue the improvement of any specific biomotor ability, a greater training volume or load is required, resulting in a cumulative increase in overall training load. Because athletes have a limited training tolerance, the increases in volume or load required to further induce changes in performance capacity eventually exceeds the athlete's ability to tolerate training (50), and ultimately, leads to a state of overtraining. This type of approach to training works well for youth and novice athletes, but may not be as beneficial for intermediate to elite athletes because these athletes require greater training stimuli in order to further develop key biomotor abilities (10, 78). Therefore, other approaches to training may be warranted for more advanced strength and power athletes (50).

Sequential Approach

The sequential approach arranges training for biomotor abilities or training targets to occur one after another in a logical pattern (figure 3.7) (10, 101).

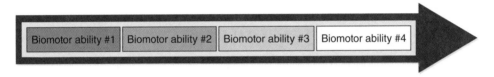

Figure 3.7 Sequential training approach.

By working specific targets sequentially, the athlete is able to undertake higher training loads and intensities in order to target a given training attribute. Strong scientific evidence supports this approach when targeting power development (46, 69, 112). Specifically, Zamparo et al. (112) and Minetti (69) suggest that the optimization of power development is achieved through a sequential pattern, which develops the muscle's cross-sectional area, improves force production capacity, and increases movement speed, resulting in increased power production capacity. Additionally, Harris et al. (46) demonstrated that training football players using a sequential training approach resulted in significantly greater increases in both power and strength measures when compared to a parallel training approach. The sequential approach to planning training serves as the foundation for the *block model of periodization* (50). While the sequential approach is a useful planning paradigm, it is possible that as the athlete moves through the sequence, detraining effects for the attributes not being trained will occur. The longer the sequence of training stimuli, the greater the chance for a detraining effect. Depending on the sport, it may be beneficial to use an approach that modulates training responses within the sequential structure.

Emphasis Approach

The emphasis, or pendulum, approach lies between the two extremes of the parallel and sequential approaches in that it incorporates aspects of both models (10).

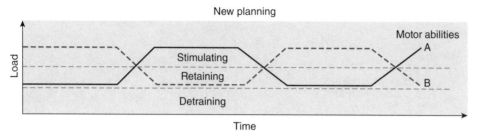

Figure 3.8   Sample emphasis model.

Reprinted, by permission, from V.M. Zatsiorsky, 1995, *Science and practice of strength training* (Champaign, IL: Human Kinetics), 126.

As noted by Zatsiorsky and Kraemer (116), this approach allows for the sequential training of various biomotor abilities with frequent intermittent changes in training emphasis. In this approach, the athlete may train several biomotor abilities (i.e., parallel approach) with varying degrees of emphasis, which changes over time (i.e., sequential approach). For example, the athlete may target the development of strength, while maintaining the ability to express power (figure 3.8).

Zatsiorsky and Kraemer (115) recommend changing the targeted biomotor ability every two weeks to optimize performance capacity. This approach seems to be particularly beneficial when attempting to maximize strength, power, and the rate of force development (115). The emphasis approach appears to be a good choice for intermediate to advanced athletes, and is best depicted in the vertical integration model presented by Francis (27).

MODELS OF PLANNING USED IN PERIODIZATION

Coaches can choose from several models to construct a periodized training plan. These models can be broken into traditional, block, and emphasis models.

Traditional Model

A central component of the traditional model is that it is a complex system that employs the parallel development of biomotor abilities (22, 90, 103). This model tends to use training structures that contain relatively limited variations in training methods and means (78, 94) that are constructed to create gradual wavelike increases in workload (63-65), which are sequenced into predetermined training structures (22). These load progressions are depicted as a ratio of the volume to the intensity of training (63). Early in the periodized training plan, the workload is primarily increased as a result of increased volumes of work and marginal increases in intensity (22). As training progresses, the volume of training decreases while the intensity of training increases. These fluctuations in intensity and volume are depicted in the figure presented by Matveyev (63, 65). This figure was, however,

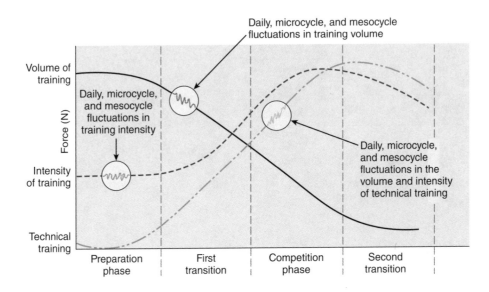

Figure 3.9 Matveyev's classic periodization model.

Reprinted by permission of Edizioni Minerva Medica from *Journal of Sports Medicine and Physical Fitness* 21: 342-351.

only meant to be a graphic illustration of the central concepts of the periodization model (figure 3.9), and was not intended to be rigidly applied to the training practices of all athletes.

The gross misinterpretation of this model has been the source for the term *linear periodization* (6, 24, 59, 60, 79) which, based on the major tenants of periodization, is not possible because central to the periodization concept is the removal of linearity. Careful inspection of Matveyev's seminal texts (63, 65) reveals that the model is in fact nonlinear and is marked by variation at several levels of the periodization hierarchy (e.g., training session, training day, microcycle, mesocycle, and macrocycle).

One of the key aspects of the traditional model is that it employs a complex parallel approach, which attempts to develop multiple biomotor abilities that are necessary for a variety of sports simultaneously (22, 90, 103). Most of the research that supports the use of this model is somewhat dated and was collected from beginner athletes (90, 103). As such, this model may not adequately address the needs of intermediate and advanced athletes (22, 103).

Block Model

Central to the block model is the idea that training needs to be prioritized and sequenced in order to allow the athlete to better manage training stressors through a more focused training approach. Strong scientific evidence supports the use of block periodization models for the development of muscular strength and maximal capacity for power generation (9, 29, 46, 77). One of the early pioneers in the development of the block model system was Dr. Anatoliy Bondarchuck, who devised a system that used three specialized mesocycle blocks for the development of throwers (12, 14, 50). These included developmental, competitive, and restoration blocks. Developmental blocks were used to increase working capacity toward maximal, while competitive blocks were focused on elevation of competitive performance. Restoration blocks were used to prepare the athlete for the next developmental block and served as transitions periods. The sequence of these blocks was predicated by the competition schedule and the athlete's responses to the training stressors (12, 14). Issurin (48, 50) proposed a model that used three basic blocks similar to those proposed by Bondarchuck (12, 14). This model used accumulation blocks to develop basic abilities (e.g., strength, endurance, movement technique), transmutation blocks to develop more specific abilities (e.g., aerobic-anaerobic or anaerobic endurance, specialized muscular endurance, power, or event-specific technique), and realization blocks to maximize performance. In its purest form, the block model uses minimal training targets in each training block and takes advantage of delayed training effects and training residuals (figure 3.10).

Emphasis Approach

The emphasis approach, as outlined by Zatsiorsky and Kraemer (116), trains several targets simultaneously with various degrees of focus, and then shifts to sequential training according to the demands of the periodized training plan. Similarly, Verkoshansky and Siff (107) give examples of integrating primary, secondary, and tertiary training emphases for a training block in their conjugated sequencing model. In this model, each block of training is vertically integrated,

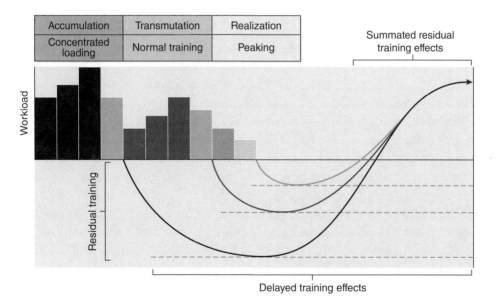

Figure 3.10 Basic block structures.

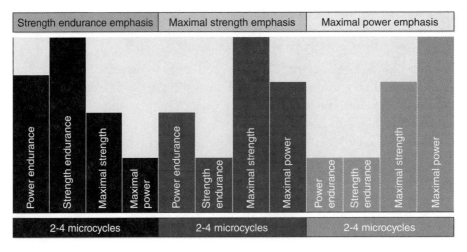

Figure 3.11 Examples of using the emphasis approach to target the development of explosive strength or power output.

meaning complementary training targets are trained to varying degrees of emphasis (emphasis approach) and horizontally sequenced (sequential approach). Horizontal sequencing then capitalizes on the training residuals and delayed training effects established in the previous block. Zatsiorsky and Kraemer (116) suggest that this model maybe ideal for the development of maximal strength, rate of force, and power in athletes in several power sports. Verkoshansky and Siff (107) give examples of how this approach can be used with athletes who are targeting the development of explosive strength or power output (figure 3.11).

FUNDAMENTALS OF POWER DEVELOPMENT

The ability to generate high power outputs is facilitated by the ability to generate high levels of force rapidly and express high contraction velocities (55). Examination of the relationship between force and velocity reveals that they are inversely related as indicated by the force–velocity curve (figure 3.12).

When examining the force–velocity curve, it is apparent that as the velocity of movement increases, the force that the muscle can produce during the concentric contraction will decrease. Because of the relationship between force and velocity, it is clear that the expression of maximal power outputs occur at compromised levels of maximal force and velocity (figure 3.13).

When targeting the optimization of power output in a training program, consider three key elements. First, *maximal strength* must be increased because it has a direct relationship with the ability to express high rates of force development and power output (3, 4, 40, 42, 69, 112). Second, a high *rate of force development* (RFD) must be achieved; this is the ability to express high forces in short periods of time and is central to the ability to express high power outputs (2, 21, 43, 67). Finally, it is

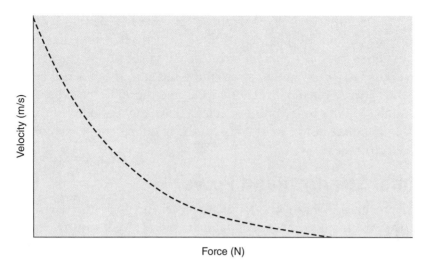

Figure 3.12   Basic force-velocity relationship.

Reprinted, by permission, from G.G. Haff and S. Nimphius, 2012, "Training principles for power," *Strength and Conditioning Journal* 34(6): 2-12.

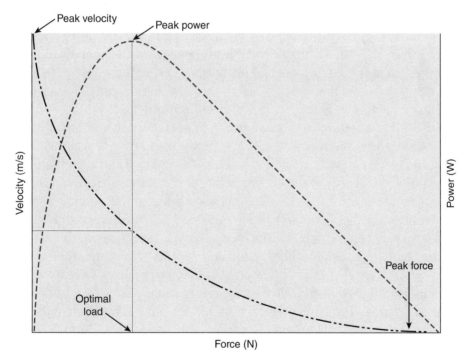

Figure 3.13   Force-velocity, force-power, velocity-power, and optimal load relationships.

Reprinted, by permission, from G.G. Haff and S. Nimphius, 2012, "Training principles for power," *Strength and Conditioning Journal* 34(6): 2-12.

important to develop the ability to express high forces as the velocity of shortening increases (40). The interplay among these elements is strong, and the athlete's overall strength serves as the main factor dictating the ability to express higher power outputs (40, 55). Within the scientific literature is evidence of the interrelationship between maximal strength, RFD, and the ability to express maximal power output (36, 42). Based on these interactions, any periodized training plan designed to optimize power must consider the development of each of these key interrelated attributes.

Maximal Strength and Power

As noted previously, one of the foundational elements in the development of power is the athlete's maximal strength (4, 40, 69, 112). Clearly, stronger athletes demonstrate a greater potential to develop higher power outputs and often express higher power outputs when compared to their weaker counterparts (4, 92). Haff and Nimphius (40) suggest that stronger people are able to generate higher forces at a higher rate when compared to weaker people (3, 42). Support for this contention can be seen in the research literature, which reports that weaker athletes who undertake resistance training that targets increasing maximal strength experience significant increases in muscular power (4, 19), which translates into improvements in athletic performance (19, 92). Once athletes have established adequate strength levels, they are then able to better capitalize on the benefits of specific power development exercises, such as plyometrics, ballistic exercises, complexes, or contrast training methods (40). In fact, it is clear that stronger athletes exhibit a greater overall responsiveness to power-based training methods (20, 40).

Based on the literature, it is clear that maximization of strength levels is a prerequisite for the development of higher power outputs. However, it is often difficult to determine what an adequate level of strength is for a given athlete or group of athletes. Based on the contemporary body of knowledge, athletes who can squat more than 2.0 × body mass express higher power outputs than their weaker counterparts (1.7 or 1.4 × body mass) (8, 92). Recent research suggests that athletes between the ages of 16 and 19 who compete in strength and power sports or team sports should be able to back squat a minimum of 2.0 × body mass (56). Additionally, when attempting to use strength–power potentiation complexes, it appears that athletes who are able to squat double their body weight are able to optimize their potentiation response for power development (82, 84). Based on this literature, Haff and Nimphius (40) suggest that a minimum back squat of 2.0 × body mass is a requirement for undertaking specialized training to optimize power output. They also suggest that strength and conditioning professionals should always include maximal strength as part of the training process for optimizing power output (40).

Rate of Force Development

The rate at which force is expressed during sporting movement is often referred to as the RFD, or explosive muscle strength (1, 67). In its most simplistic form, RFD is determined from the slope of the force–time curve (108) (figure 3.14). One can calculate the RFD in a variety of ways, including the peak value in a predetermined sampling window and specific time bands, such as the slope of 0-200 meters per second (ms) (41). Typically, contraction times of 50-250 ms are associated with jumping, sprinting, and change-of-direction movements. With short contraction times, it is unlikely that maximal forces can be developed, and it has been reported that it may take >300 ms to generate maximal forces (1, 95, 97). With this in mind, several authors recommend ballistic exercises performed with light loads as a method to optimize RFD and subsequently the overall power output (21, 75).

When examining the scientific literature, it is clear that performing resistance training exercises with heavy loads results in an increase in maximal strength (21, 75) and RFD in weaker or untrained people (62). While training with heavy loads increases most athletes' strength reserve and can positively affect their RFD, it is likely that explosive or ballistic exercises may be necessary to optimize RFD in stronger, more experienced athletes (21, 43). Based on this phenomenon, Haff and Nimphius (40) suggest that varying the training foci has the potential to affect various parts of the force–time curve (figure 3.15) and force–velocity curve (figure 3.16).

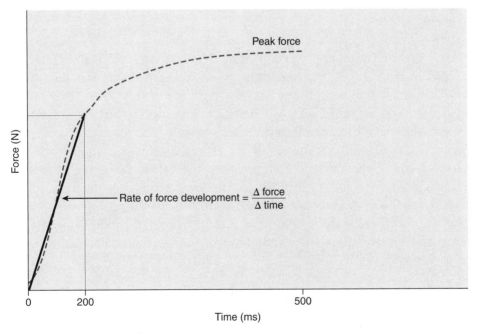

Figure 3.14 Isometric force-time curve.

Reprinted, by permission, from G.G. Haff and S. Nimphius, 2012, "Training principles for power," *Strength and Conditioning Journal* 34(6): 2-12.

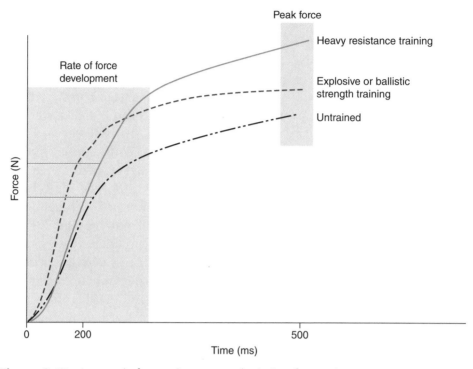

Figure 3.15 Isometric force–time curve depicting force–time curve responses to training.

Reprinted, by permission, from G.G. Haff and S. Nimphius, 2012, "Training principles for power," *Strength and Conditioning Journal* 34(6): 2-12.

Heavy resistance training and explosive or ballistic strength training have the potential to increase an untrained athlete's maximal strength and RFD (figure 3.15). Conversely, ballistic training does not increase maximal strength, but results in a greater increase in the RFD when compared to heavy resistance training in stronger athletes. When examining the force–velocity relationship, it is clear that heavy resistance training results in increases in the velocity of movement at the high-force end of the curve (figure 3.16b), while ballistic movements result in increases in the velocity of movement at the low-force end of the force-velocity curve (figure 3.16c). It is clear that mixed methods that target high-velocity and high-force movements are necessary to exert a more global effect on the force-velocity relationship (figure 3.16a and figure 3.16d) and ultimately increase RFD and power output (40).

PLANNING TRAINING AND POWER DEVELOPMENT

When looking at the periodization literature, one can choose from several planning models to target the maximization of power. The first approach is the use of

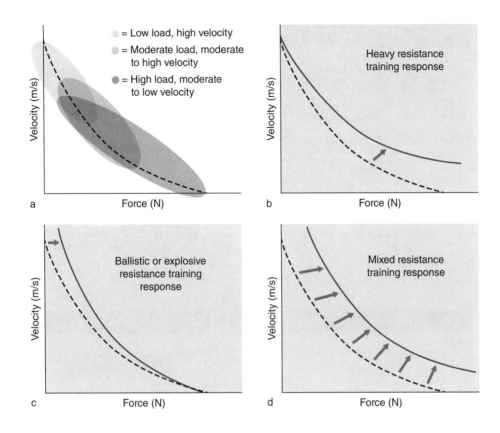

Figure 3.16 Potential training interventions that affect the force–velocity curve.

Reprinted, by permission, from G.G. Haff and S. Nimphius, 2012, "Training principles for power," *Strength and Conditioning Journal* 34(6): 2-12.

the traditional approach in which the athlete attempts to develop all key biomotor abilities in a parallel approach (figure 3.17).

In this approach, equal attention is given to each of the key attributes across the entire annual training plan. As noted earlier, this approach may work for novice or youth athletes, but it is probably not the ideal approach for more advanced athletes. More advanced athletes may require other more advanced planning models in order to fully maximize the development of power.

The second approach to the development of power is the sequential model of periodization. Strong scientific support demonstrates that by dedicating specific time periods to a target, key attributes can be developed in a sequential fashion, resulting in the optimization of power-generating capacity. Based on the model proposed by Zamparo et al. (112) and Minetti (69), a coach could use an approach that sequentially targets muscle hypertrophy, maximal strength, strength-power, and then power development (figure 3.18).

This model is similar to the approach presented by Stone, O'Bryant, and Gar-hammer (93) in their seminal paper on periodization for strength training. In this

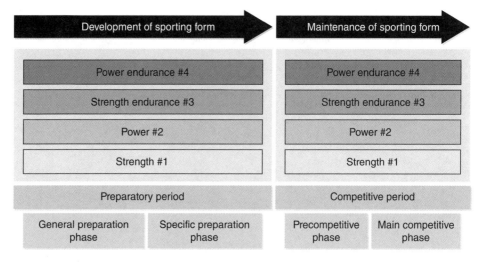

Figure 3.17 Parallel approach to power development.

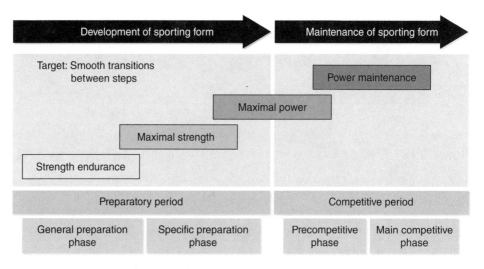

Figure 3.18 Sequential approach to power development.

model, distinctive training targets were sequentially developed across a 12-week training plan, resulting in a significant increase in the capacity to generate maximal power. This approach appears to work well for intermediate to advanced athletes.

The third model of planning one could use is the emphasis approach. In this approach, the main training factors are vertically integrated and horizontally sequenced (figure 3.19).

Complementary training factors are trained at various levels of emphasis, and then are sequenced across a series of mesocycle blocks to optimize the transfer of key adaptive responses to power development. At the same time, training stimuli are supplied to minimize the detraining effects that may occur in sequential models. As with the sequential model, this approach works well for intermediate to advanced athletes.

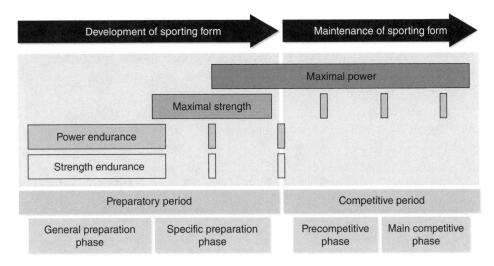

Figure 3.19 Emphasis approach to power development.

PROGRAMMING AND POWER DEVELOPMENT

Once the overall periodization plan and the training model are established, a training program can be developed. Central to programming is establishing the intensity of training, set structures employed, types of exercise used, strength-power potentiation complexes, and exercise order.

Intensity of Training

A lot of research has been conducted to determine the *optimal load* for power development when performing resistance training. It has been suggested that the use of the optimal load is an effective methodology for improving power output (21, 54, 55, 68, 70, 99, 100, 109). However, few studies actually support this contention (54, 68, 70, 109), and several studies suggest that training with heavy loads (19, 47) or mixed loads (99, 100) produces superior enhancements in power output.

Training at the optimal load, while conceptually sound, appears to be flawed because the current body of knowledge indicates that many athletes require the ability to express high power outputs under loaded conditions (4, 5). In fact, in sports like rugby league, a critical differentiator of performance is the athlete's overall strength levels and ability to express high power outputs under loaded conditions (4, 5). For these types of athletes, the use of the optimal load to develop power will result in a muted ability to improve strength levels (19, 47, 68, 99, 100), which is detrimental to these athletes. Therefore, it may be warranted to use training loads in excess of the optimal load in order to improve the ability to express high power outputs under loaded conditions. In support of this contention, Moss et al. (70) report that training with heavier loads (>80% of 1RM) enhances power development under loaded conditions (>60% of 1RM) when compared to training with moderate to low training loads (<30% of 1RM). When working with athletes who must express high power outputs in loaded conditions (e.g., rugby league, rugby union, American football), it is critical that strength development be a central component of training.

Many athletes must produce force against external sources of resistance and therefore need to train at a variety of training loads in order to develop power more globally in a variety of conditions. This becomes important when athletes must develop power in unloaded conditions such as sprinting and are often required to make large changes of direction, which magnifies the load that the athlete must resist or move against (40). Additionally, athletes must also produce forces against external resistances in activities such as tackling or during rowing, where high forces are met continually during performance. Because athletes encounter a continuum of loads in sport, it is imperative to expose them to a variety of loads in training (40). Therefore, to optimize the continuum of power needed in sport, the strength and conditioning professional should adopt a mixed-methods model of training that works the athlete's ability to generate power across the entire range of the force–velocity profile (40, 55).

One strategy for employing a mixed-methods approach is to use a variety of training loads when constructing the training program (40). For example, the back squat typically uses higher loads (>75% of 1RM) to develop lower body strength. However, it can also be used with lighter loads (e.g., 30%-70% of 1RM) to develop power (figure 3.20).

An additional consideration in power-based training is the use of the warm-up set as a key contributor to performing training at various parts of the force–velocity relationship (40). For example, if an athlete were using the back squat to develop lower body strength with loads of 80%-85% of 1RM, he or she would perform a series of lower-loaded warm-up sets and, if performed explosively, could be used to develop power (57). Lifting submaximal and maximal loads as quickly as possible in an explosive manner provides a greater potential for developing power across a range of training loads even when using exercises that are traditionally reserved for strength development (40, 57).

Set Structures

When examining the ability to develop power, the structure of the set can play an integral role in developing power within a given exercise. Traditional set structures, in which reps are performed in a continuous manner without rest between repetitions, result in a reduction in the power output achieved in each repetition in the set (44). For example, Hardee et al. (44) report that across a set of 6 repetitions in the power clean, there is a 15.7% reduction in power output from rep 1 to 6. Additionally, Gorostiage et al. (30) report a 7%-20% reduction in average peak power during the leg press when traditional sets of 5 were used and a 35%-45% reduction when sets of 10 repetitions were performed. Interestingly, the higher-

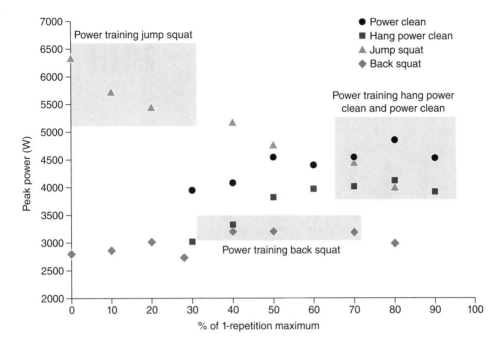

Figure 3.20 Resistance training exercises and power zones.

Reprinted, by permission, from G.G. Haff and S. Nimphius, 2012, "Training principles for power," *Strength and Conditioning Journal* 34(6): 2-12.

volume sets depicted a greater reduction in ATP and phosphocreatine, while a greater increase in lactate was demonstrated (30), which may partially explain why there was a reduction in power output across the set structure. Collectively, these data suggest that when attempting to maximize power output, sets of less than 6 reps are needed when using traditional set structures to optimize the development of power. To maximize power outputs during training, other resistance training set strategies, such as cluster sets, may be warranted, especially if higher-volume work is targeted (35, 39).

The cluster set as defined by Haff et al. (35, 39) is a set structure that applies a short rest interval (15-45 s) between individual repetitions or small groupings of repetitions in order to induce partial recovery and maximize the velocity and power of the movement (figure 3.21). Hardee et al. (44) noted that performing power cleans with 80% of 1RM using cluster sets with 20 s rest between repetitions resulted in only a 5.5% reduction in power output across 6 repetitions. They compared this to a traditional set that demonstrated a 15.7% decrease. When the rest interval used in the cluster set was extended to 40 s, the reduction in power output was only 3.3%. The increased power output that occurs by extending the interrepetition rest interval to 30-40 s appears to capitalize on the ability to partially replenish phosphocreatine and ATP during these recovery periods (35, 39).

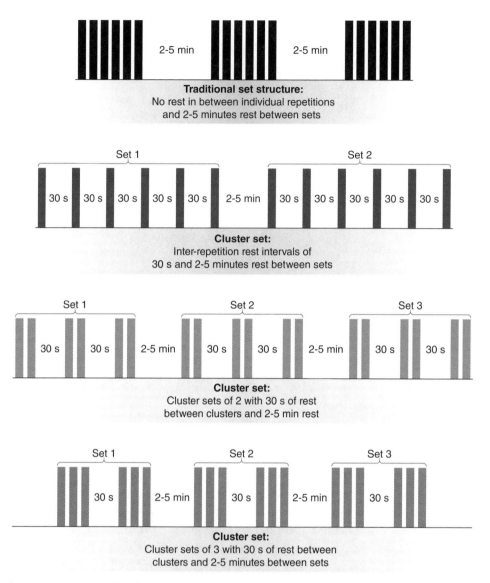

Figure 3.21 Sample cluster set structures used for power development.

When structuring cluster sets, Haff et al. (35) suggest three basic variants can be used: the standard, the undulating, and the ascending cluster sets (table 3.2). The standard cluster set uses a loading scheme in which every repetition is performed with the exact same load and only the interrepetition rest interval is manipulated. An alternative approach is to use an undulating or ascending cluster set, manipulating the repetition load and the interrepetition rest interval. During the undulating set structure, the load increases in a pyramid fashion, while the ascending cluster set increases the load of each repetition performed in the set. An additional cluster set modification could be the manipulation of the number of repetitions performed. For example, a cluster set of 6 repetitions

Table 3.2 Sample Cluster Set Structures for the Power Snatch

Type of cluster	Sets	×	Repetitions	Sample structure for cluster set repetition loading (weight[kg]/ repetition[#])					Interrepetition rest interval (s)
Standard	1-3	×	5/1	106/1	106/1	106/1	106/1	106/1	30
	1-3	×	6/2	106/2	106/2	106/2			30
	1-3	×	5/3, 2	102/3	102/2				30
Undulating	1-3	×	5/1	103/1	106/1	113/2	106/2	103/2	30
	1-3	×	6/2	104/2	110/2	104/2			30
Ascending	1-3	×	5/1	98/1	103/1	105/1	110/1	113/1	30
	1-3	×	6/2	100/2	106/2	113/2			30

5/1 = 5 total repetitions broken into 5 clusters of 1; 6/2 = 6 total repetitions broken into 3 clusters of 2; 5/3,2 = 5 total repetitions broken into 1 cluster of 3 and 1 cluster of 2.

All weights based on max power snatch of 125 kg (106 kg = 85% of 1RM).

Each set has an average intensity of 106 kg or 85% of 1RM.

could be performed with rest between individual repetitions (6/1) or between pairs of repetitions (6/2) or between groups of 3 repetitions (6/3) with varying rest intervals. By varying the repetitions and rest intervals between reps or clusters of repetitions, different aspects of power may be developed. Regardless of the cluster set structures employed, the rest interval between sets is typically 2-5 min when attempting to maximize power (37).

When contextualized to the periodized training plan, cluster sets seem to offer their best benefits during the specific preparatory phases of the annual training plan (80). For example, Roll and Omer (80) recommend using cluster sets with the clean and bench press exercises during the specific preparatory phase (e.g., strength–power phase) of the annual training plan when working with American football players. Similarly, Haff et al. (35, 39) suggest that cluster sets are ideally suited for the specific preparatory phase when maximizing power development is a central training target.

Types of Exercises Used

When developing a resistance training program that is in line with the periodization and planning goals, the actual training exercises selected play a key role in effectively developing power. Haff and Nimphius (40) suggest that a mixed-methods approach is essential when attempting to develop various parts of the force–velocity curve. Training exercises can be broken into several distinct categories, including shock or reactive-strength, speed-strength, strength-speed, maximal-strength, and supramaximal-strength methods. Each of these methods develops different aspects of the force–velocity curve and, as such, affect power development in different ways. For example, shock or reactive-strength training maximizes the engagement of the stretch-shortening cycle and generally requires the athlete to couple an eccentric and concentric muscle action in an explosive manner. The best example of a reactive-strength activity is high-level plyometrics such as a drop or depth jump from a box, requiring the athlete to rapidly jump vertically after contacting the ground (chapter 6). Speed-strength training enhances the RFD and in general has a high power output (94). On the other hand, strength-speed training targets the development of the RFD, but tends to use heavier loads. These loads however are not as high as those used to develop maximal or supramaximal strength. Some of these methods are introduced here but will also be discussed in more detail in chapter 8.

For example, ballistic methods could use plyometric activities, which target the low-force high-velocity portion of the force–time curve (40). Strength-speed methods could use moderate loads of 50%-85% of 1RM with exercises such as the clean pull or power clean to develop power across a wide range of the force–velocity curve. Maximal-strength methods would use loads >85% of 1RM and use a variety of exercises, such as the back squat to develop loaded power output at the high-force end of the force–velocity curve. Each exercise has a different power profile and can be used in different ways depending on loading to affect the development of specific strength and power attributes depending on how they are employed in the training program.

When examining the power profile of a variety of exercises, it is apparent that each exercise has a different power profile (see figure 3.22). For example, weightlifting movements (e.g., snatch, clean and jerk) and their derivatives (e.g., clean pull,

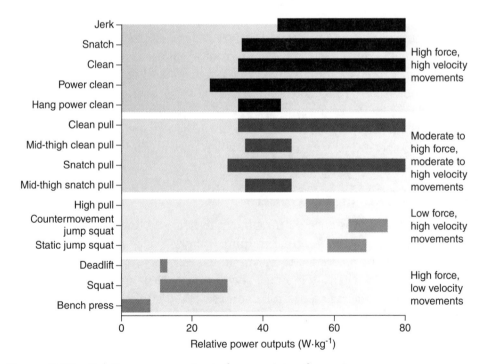

Figure 3.22 Relative power outputs for a variety of exercises.

Reprinted, by permission, from G.G. Haff and S. Nimphius, 2012, "Training principles for power," *Strength and Conditioning Journal* 34(6): 2-12.

snatch pull, and push press) offer the ability to develop large amounts of power across a wide range of the force–velocity relationship (chapter 7).

Conversely, powerlifting exercises (i.e., squat, bench press, and deadlift) produce very little power. Therefore, they affect the high-force portion of the force–velocity curve.

Strength–Power Potentiation Complexes

Recently, interest has grown in the use of strength–power potentiation complexes in which previous muscular contractions are used to acutely increase the production of strength and power in subsequent exercises (85-88). Strength–power potentiation complexes contain a heavy-load conditioning activity followed by a high-power performance activity. Typically, the time frame between the conditioning and performance activity can range from 4-10 min, but is most typically about 5 min. Examination of the various conditioning activities used for lower body strength–power potentiation complexes reveals that either the back squat or the power clean is used (88). However, recent research by Seitz et al. (88) suggests that the power clean results in significantly greater sprint performance when compared to the back squat. Regardless of the exercise protocol used, the general format of the conditioning activity typically uses heavy-load or ascending protocols that go up to ~90% of the athlete's 1RM (table 3.3).

Table 3.3 Sample Strength–Power Potentiating Complexes

Potentiation-inducing activity	Recovery time (min)	Performance activity
Heavy-load squat 3 reps at 90% of 1RM	4-5	40 m sprint
Heavy-load power clean 3 reps at 90% of 1RM	7	20 m sprint
Heavy-load squat 3 reps at 90% of 1RM	7	20 m sprint
Heavy-load squats 3 reps at 90% of 1RM	3-6	Squat jump
Ascending squat 5 reps at 30% 1RM 4 reps at 50% 1RM 3 reps at 70% 1RM	4-5	40 m sprint
Ascending squat 5 reps at 30% 1RM 3 reps at 50% 1RM 3 reps at 70% 1RM 3 reps at 90% 1RM	4-5	5 horizontal plyometric jumps
Ascending squat 2 reps at 20% 1RM 2 reps at 40% 1RM 2 reps at 60% 1RM 2 reps at 80% 1RM 2 reps at 90% 1RM	4-5	Vertical jump

Based on Seitz et al. (84), Seitz et al. (88), Gourgoulis et al. (31), McBride et al. (66), Ruben et al. (82), and Yetter et al. (111).

When closely examining the use of strength–power potentiation complexes, it appears that the ability to maximize the performance gain from the conditioning activity is largely affected by the athlete's overall strength, the exercise used in the conditioning exercise, the time window after the conditioning activity, and the exercise used during the conditioning activity (84, 98).

When programming strength–power potentiation complexes in a periodized training plan, consider where in the program these are best suited. Typically, these activities are used in phases that optimize power output or transition from maximal strength development to power development. They are typically used in the specific preparatory phase (80,85). However, because strength–power potentiation complexes are mixed-methods activities that target strength and power simultaneously, they may be useful during the precompetitive and main competitive phases of the annual training plan. This modality is discussed in more detail in chapter 8.

Exercise Order

When constructing a training program, most exercise order guidelines suggest that power exercises be performed before core and assistance exercises (37). This order is effective because power exercises often require more effort, skill, and focus than multijoint core exercises and single-joint assistance exercises, and thus should be performed when fresh. While this strategy is excellent, it may not be the best approach for stronger, more developed athletes because they may need more advanced training structures to maximize performance gains. Another way to organize a training program is through ascending or descending workouts (96). Ascending workouts start with shock or reactive-strength exercises, followed by ballistic, strength-speed, and heavy load strength exercises (table 3.4). Ascending workouts increase force application and reduce the velocity of movement across training sessions.

Conversely, descending workouts reverse this order, starting with heavy load strength exercises and ending with shock or ballistic exercises (table 3.5). By reversing the order of the session, the athlete progresses from higher- to lower-force activities, while increasing movement velocity.

Both the ascending and descending methods allow develop various portions of the force–velocity curve and can affect power development across a variety of loading structures.

Table 3.4 *Sample Ascending Workout*

Exercise	Sets	×	Reps	Load (% 1RM)	Focus
Depth jump	3	×	5	0	Shock or reactive-strength
Jump squat	3	×	5	0-30	Ballistic
Power clean	3	×	5	75-85	Strength-speed
Back squat	3	×	5	80-85	Strength

Table 3.5 Sample Descending Workout

Exercise	Sets	×	Reps	Load (% 1RM)	Focus
Back squat	3	×	5	80-85	Strength
Power clean	3	×	5	75-85	Strength-speed
Jump squat	3	×	5	0-30	Ballistic
Depth jump	3	×	5	0	Shock or reactive-strength

CONCLUSION

Based on the contemporary body of scientific knowledge, periodized training plans are an essential component of the development of athletic performance. Once a multiyear or annual training plan is established, one can plan the organization of the training structures and determine which training methods to include in the program for developing power. A parallel planning structure may be an adequate tool for guiding the training process of novice athletes. However, for intermediate to advanced athletes, sequential or emphasis models may provide a superior training stimulus for the maximization of both strength and power. Regardless of the planning structure used, it is essential that the strength and conditioning professional understands that strength is the foundation from which power is built and that the development of strength should always be part of the training process. When targeting strength and power development, a mixed training model approach is necessary. Training structures, such as strength–power potentiation complexes and cluster sets, can be useful when constructing training interventions. Additionally, ascending and descending structures can be useful components of a training plan to maximize power development.

CHAPTER 4

Power Training for Different Populations

N. Travis Triplett,
PhD, CSCS,*D

Rhodri S. Lloyd,
PhD, CSCS,*D

Many strength and conditioning professionals work with a range of ages and abilities among their clientele. This chapter presents power training guidelines for populations that have distinctive characteristics and may require modification of standard training protocols in order to maximize training effects and minimize risk of injury. When designing programs to improve power, it is important to understand power training in the context of both young, developing athletes and older people who may have a variety of complicating factors in their medical history.

TRAINING YOUTH POPULATIONS

Whether a child or an adolescent is involved in competitive sports, engages in recreational physical activity, or simply needs to perform daily physical tasks, the ability to produce maximal neuromuscular power is an essential physical capacity. The capacity to produce high quantities of neuromuscular power is a requirement for dynamic sporting performance (30) because higher power outputs are typically characteristic of superior sporting success (57). Muscular power is also an important physical attribute for force absorption when rapidly changing direction or dealing with unanticipated movements (65). Therefore, both children and adolescents should engage in training methods that promote the development of neuromuscular power.

The most common training modality for developing neuromuscular power is some form of resistance training. Resistance training is a specialized method of training whereby a person works against a wide range of resistive loads applied through the use of body weight, weight machines, free weights (barbells and dumbbells), elastic bands, and medicine balls (40). Despite previous concerns regarding its safety, resistance training is now recognized as a safe and effective vehicle for developing muscular strength and power in children and adolescents and should serve as an essential part of daily physical activity for all youth (40). Practitioners who plan, deliver, and guide athletic development programs for youth should possess a sound understanding of pediatric exercise science, a recognized strength and conditioning qualification (e.g., certified strength and conditioning specialist), a background in pedagogy (i.e., the method and practice of teaching), and an ability to communicate with youth of different ages and abilities.

Assessing Power in Youth Populations

A wide of range of equipment now exists to assess the kinetics and kinematics of isometric and dynamic athletic performance, with the most predominant testing protocols involving various forms of jumping, sprinting, or projection (51) (see chapter 2). Measurement tools previously used to assess neuromuscular power in youth populations include force plates and linear position transducers (15, 27), mobile contact mats (43), motion analysis systems (37), and isokinetic dynamometry (11). Another piece of equipment often used to determine short-term power output in youth is the cycle ergometer, on which children and adolescents have often been assessed for performance using the Wingate anaerobic test (2). Regardless of the testing equipment or protocol used, the manner in which these tests are administered is critical. Youth require familiarization sessions, clear and child-friendly instructions, and, wherever possible, child-sized equipment.

While studies have used the Wingate anaerobic cycle test to assess short-term power output, performance is less dependent on neuromuscular coordination and arguably more reliant on biochemical endurance (50). Consequently, in order to determine how two children compare in terms of neuromuscular power or in order to assess the effectiveness of a training intervention, practitioners are encouraged to use test protocols that require single maximal efforts at submaximal velocities and loads. The test protocol that appears most often in the pediatric literature and that is used most frequently by practitioners is the vertical jump (45). As stated in chapter 2, using a force plate, peak power is quantified from the ground reaction forces and velocity of center of mass displacement, whereas peak power can be calculated indirectly by jump height and body mass using a contact mat. Because of their relative ease of administration, vertical-jump protocols are routinely used within the pediatric setting, with practitioners favoring lower-cost contact mats or similar jump-and-reach equipment over more costly equipment such as force plates. Vertical-jump performance has been used to track motor skill development in school age youth (25, 31), assess physical performance in young athletes (48), and monitor the effectiveness of training interventions (47) and is commonly used as a component of talent identification protocols in sport (69).

Research shows that muscular power increases in a nonlinear fashion throughout childhood and adolescence, with both boys and girls of all ages and maturity levels able to show improvement as a result of growth and maturation alone (7). This is an important factor for researchers and practitioners to consider as they plan and deliver strength and conditioning programs, because growth and maturity-related increases in neuromuscular power may be misinterpreted as training-induced adaptations. Consequently, practitioners should understand the typical gains in performance expected as a result of growth and maturation in addition to the measurement error associated with the testing equipment used in order to confidently determine meaningful changes in performance associated with training.

Natural Development of Neuromuscular Power in Youth

The natural development of neuromuscular power mirrors that of muscular strength, which is unsurprising given the close association between the two physical qualities (77). Indeed, much like muscular strength, natural gains in neuromuscular power (as measured by performance in standing long jump) have been shown to occur in prepubertal children between the ages of 5 and 10 years (9). Maturation of the central nervous system is typically responsible for the adaptations seen in neuromuscular power during childhood. Specifically, the ability to activate and coordinate motor units and the increased neural myelination improve neural drive through this stage of development (23). A secondary natural "spurt" in neuromuscular power then appears to commence approximately 18 months before peak height velocity (approximately 10.5 years for girls and 12.5 years boys), with peak gains typically occurring 6-12 months after peak height velocity (6). Peak height velocity refers to the maximum rate of growth during the adolescent growth curve. In addition to the continuing maturation of the nervous system, adolescence is associated with structural and architectural changes in contractile tissue, which ultimately increases the capacity to generate force. Proliferations in hormonal concentrations (including testosterone, growth hormone, and insulin-like growth factor) mediate changes in muscle size, muscle pennation angle, and further motor unit differentiation (78).

The ability to produce high levels of muscular power depends on the type of muscular action involved, and research has demonstrated that when a muscle uses a stretch-shortening cycle (SSC), it can produce greater power outputs than an isolated concentric contraction (36). Owing to the dynamics of sport and physical activity, rarely is a concentric action used in isolation; therefore, it is important to consider how the ability of young children to effectively use the SSC changes as they mature. Research shows that the development of the SSC is nonlinear, with periods of accelerated adaptation for a range of measures of SSC function reported for age ranges indicative of pre- and postpeak height velocity (44). Additionally, the same researchers examined the manner in which the neural regulation of SSC function changes in children of different maturity groups and showed that as children become older and more mature, they become more reliant on feed-forward mechanisms (preactivation) to regulate cyclical high-speed activities that produce a high rate of force, such as submaximal or maximal hopping in place (46). Feed-forward activity reflects involuntary anticipatory muscle activity prior to the observation of any spinal or supraspinal reflexive activity.

Trainability of Neuromuscular Power in Youth

Research shows that traditional resistance training, ballistic exercises, plyometrics, and weightlifting are the most commonly used forms of resistance training to develop neuromuscular power (13). While literature examining the interaction between growth, maturation, and the trainability of neuromuscular power remains scarce, several studies show that both children and adolescents are able to increase this physical quality following exposure to appropriate resistance-based training interventions. Within the pediatric literature, research shows that traditional resistance training (52), plyometrics (47), weightlifting (11), explosive strength training (28), and combined training (83) are all safe and effective means of enhancing various indices of neuromuscular power. Resistance training has also been shown to increase insulin sensitivity in obese youth because the training mode can increase both the size and recruitment of fast-twitch muscle fibers (74).

Because there is little evidence of hypertrophic adaptations in children, resistance training–induced gains in neuromuscular power during childhood is likely determined by changes in the nervous system (5). Conversely, training-induced gains in neuromuscular power during adolescence typically reflect not only adaptations to the nervous system but also structural and architectural properties (53). More research is required to examine the specific mechanisms that mediate training-induced gains in neuromuscular power in youth, especially those that underpin long-term adaptations across different stages of maturation.

A fundamental relationship exists between muscular strength and neuromuscular power. Evidence shows that people with higher strength levels have a greater capacity to produce power (13). Given its multiple health and performance benefits and its ability to reduce the risk of injury, resistance training should form an integral part of any youth-based strength and conditioning program (40). Practitioners should ensure that all children and adolescents are provided with developmentally appropriate training strategies to develop sound movement mechanics while simultaneously increasing muscular strength levels (40). In combination, movement competency and muscular strength will serve as the foundations for a robust system through which high levels of muscular power can be produced and attenuated during whole-body dynamic activities. The emphasis on muscular strength and movement competency is especially prudent considering the negative trends in muscular strength levels and motor fitness of modern-day youth (12, 70). Because of the increased sedentariness of children (79) and the fact that children are less capable of maximally recruiting their high-threshold Type II motor units (18), it is highly probable that in most cases simply by focusing on increasing movement competency and muscular strength capacities, practitioners will be able to indirectly increase neuromuscular power.

Researchers have examined the effects of a 2-year resistance training program on strength performance in youth soccer players and have shown that the magnitude of strength gains increases with age (35). Long-term exposure to periodized resistance training resulted in relative strength levels being 0.7 × body weight in 11- 12-year-olds, 1.5 × body weight in 13- 15-year-olds, and 2.0 × body weight in 16- 19-year-olds (35). In a separate study, the same group of researchers showed that after 2 years of strength training, 13-, 15-, and 17-year-old soccer players simultaneously improved 1RM squat strength (100%-300%) and sprinting speed (3%-5%), which was used as a surrogate measure of power (71).

Not all youth wish to engage in competitive sports; therefore, practitioners should not base strength and power training prescription on data from homogenous populations (e.g., elite youth soccer players). Research has examined the effectiveness of integrative neuromuscular training interventions on the health- and skill-related measures of fitness in 7-year-old school-age children (21). The study showed that children were able to make significant gains in curl-up and push-up performance (increased muscular strength and endurance) and also long jump and single-leg hop performance (increased neuromuscular power) by following an 8-week, twice-weekly (15-min sessions) training program (21). A follow-up study showed that after an 8-week detraining period, training-induced gains in curl-up and single-leg hop performance (muscular strength and endurance) were maintained, while those for long jump performance (neuromuscular power) significantly decreased (22). This might suggest that muscular strength is easier to maintain in children, while neuromuscular power capacities require more frequent stimuli to prevent detraining.

Improvements in muscular power have also been shown in school-age youth who followed a 4-week plyometric training program (47). This study showed that 12- and 15-year-old boys were able to significantly improve SSC function, while 9-year-olds were also able to show improvements, albeit not significantly. This may highlight an age-dependent response to plyometric training and may indicate that younger children possibly require a different amount of training to elicit similar gains, such as those their more mature peers experience. Conversely, it could simply suggest that training-induced adaptation takes longer to materialize in younger children, which supports the notion of a long-term approach to training for athletic development in youth. Cumulatively, these studies show that both children and adolescents can make resistance training gains in neuromuscular power, that youth can make improvements in neuromuscular power as a result of increasing their muscular strength capacities, and that training-induced gains in neuromuscular power may diminish at a faster rate than muscular strength in youth.

Translating the Science Into Program Design

When designing training programs for children or adolescents, progression should be based primarily on the technical competency of the person. Practitioners should also consider the training age of the children or adolescents (55), which reflects their relative experience (e.g. number of years) of formalized training, and potentially, the type of training to which they have been exposed. Coaches should also be aware of the biological maturation of the person because stages of development are characterized by unique physiological adaptations that may affect the design of the training program (42). Because of the inherent variations of the timing, tempo, and magnitude of maturation, chronological age should not determine training prescriptions for youths. Psychosocial maturity should also be taken into account when designing a program to meet the individual needs of the child (40). For example, an inexperienced and introverted child lacking confidence may need simpler exercises, more conservative progressions, and a greater degree of patience than an experienced, confident, and extroverted adolescent. The following case studies demonstrate how training prescription is altered in accord with the individual needs of children or adolescents with varying degrees of experience and technical competency.

Case Study 1: Child With No Training Experience and Low Technical Competency

When a young child is first exposed to a formalized strength and conditioning program, it is unlikely the child will be able to demonstrate competency in a range of motor skills. Consequently, initial focus should be directed toward developing a diverse range of motor skills that will benefit overall athleticism (figure 4.1). Before trying to develop muscular power, coaches should look to increase muscular strength levels because an untrained child with low technical competency will be a considerable distance from his or her ceiling potential of force-producing capacities. Therefore, in addition to training motor skills, base levels of muscular strength should also be trained during the early stages of the training program to enable the expression of higher levels of neuromuscular power. This approach should also provide a robust and highly coordinated neuromuscular system that youth can use to withstand the reactive and unpredictable forces typically experienced within free play, sports, or recreational physical activity. A sample training session for an inexperienced child with low technical competency is provided in table 4.1.

Children with low technical competency should also be exposed to a range of activities that enable the simultaneous development of other fitness qualities, such as coordination, speed, power, agility, and flexibility (41). This is because of the heightened neural plasticity associated with childhood and the accompanying trainability of neuromuscular qualities (5). While the development of neuromuscular power is critical for sport performance, recreational physical activity, and

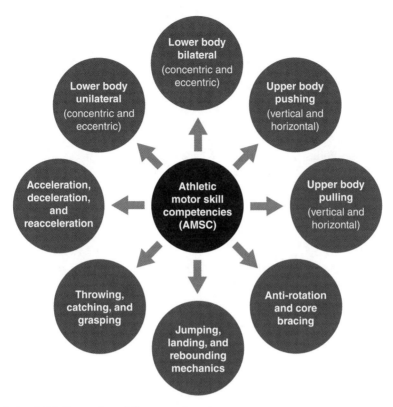

Figure 4.1 Athletic motor skill competencies.

From J.A. Moody, F. Naclerio, P. Green, and R.S. Lloyd, 2013, Motor skill development in youths. In *Strength and conditioning for young athletes: Science and application*, edited by R.S. Lloyd and J.L. Oliver (Oxon: Routledge), 53. Reproduced by permission of Taylor & Francis Books UK.

general health and well-being, taking a broader approach to athletic development in youth is important because of the inherent trainability of all fitness components at all stages of development (41). Consequently, strength and conditioning coaches should not focus on one or two measures of fitness, but should rather provide complementary training activities that develop a wide range of fitness components.

Additionally, a varied and holistic approach to athletic development is necessary from a pedagogical perspective in order to keep training sessions fun, interesting, and motivating for the young child (39). Practitioners should remember that many activities that children engage in on the playground (e.g., hop scotch) present opportunities for power training and that child-friendly activities that might not reflect the traditional training modes (e.g., advanced plyometrics or weightlifting) can still be effective in developing neuromuscular power.

In terms of developing neuromuscular power, practitioners should view childhood as an opportunity to lay the foundation of general athleticism that will then enable youth to participate in more advanced training strategies as they become more experienced. For example, a major goal for practitioners working with a

Table 4.1 Sample Training Session for a Child With No Training Experience and Low Technical Competency

Phase	Exercise	Description	Volume (sets × reps)	Intensity	Rest (s)
Fun warm-up	Animal shapes warm-up games	Child moves around the floor in multiple directions using various animal shapes (e.g. bear, crab or seal).	4 × 30 seconds	Bodyweight	30
Bodyweight Management	Deadbugs	Child lays on back with the arms extended towards the ceiling and the hips, knees, and ankles at 90 degrees. Then, the child extends one leg and one arm asynchronously and then returns them to center.	2 × 10 (each side)	Bodyweight	30
	Inchworms	Child places the hands in front of the feet, and then walks the hands out as far as possible while maintaining torso control. Then, the child the walks feet into the hands.	2 × 8	Bodyweight	30
	Dish-to-arch rolls	Child rolls from a dish position to and arch and back to a dish position without the feet, hands or head touching the floor.	2 × 8 (each side)	Bodyweight	30
	Front support walks	The first child adopts a front support position, while a partner supports the ankles and the shins. Then, the first child moves around the floor in multiple directions and maintains torso control.	2 × 10 m	Bodyweight	45

Phase	Exercise	Description	Volume (sets × reps)	Intensity	Rest (s)
Main	30 cm (11.8 inches) box jumps		3 × 4	Bodyweight	45
	Resistance band overhead squat		3 × 6	Bodyweight plus band tension	60
	Push-ups		3 × 6	Bodyweight	45
	Band standing rows		3 × 6	Bodyweight plus band tension	45

child with low technical competency might be to develop the ability to jump and land effectively. This should be viewed as a critical athletic motor skill that is required for a range of activities, for example, plyometric training. Over time, and as technical competency and muscular strength increase, the child can challenge this movement pattern through a higher plyometric training stimulus that provides a greater eccentric stress (e.g., drop jumps or bounding). Another example could be in the development of weightlifting ability, whereby childhood should be viewed as an opportunity to develop basic motor skills that will help in the execution of full weightlifting movements and their derivatives as technical competency improves.

Case Study 2: Technically Competent Adolescent With 6 Years of Training Experience

When a child has engaged with formalized training during childhood, adolescence can serve as an ideal opportunity to build on existing levels of neuromuscular fitness. Developmentally appropriate training can be prescribed to work synergistically with the heightened hormonal concentrations that result from puberty. This enables the adolescent to achieve greater neural, structural, and architectural adaptations. Consequently, technically competent adolescents with a sound training age should be able to generate greater force outputs at higher velocities, thus enhancing their ability to produce high levels of neuromuscular power. As part of their athletic development program, technically competent adolescents of an appropriate training age should incorporate a variety of resistance training modes to develop neuromuscular power, using higher intensities (e.g., greater external loads or movement velocities), more sophisticated training strategies (e.g., complex training or cluster training), or more advanced technical demands (e.g., accentuated plyometric training, weightlifting derivatives) or a combination of these variables. Practitioners should regularly revisit the adolescent's motor skill competency, regardless of his or her training history, in order to prevent technical deficiencies over time stemming from sudden growth spurts, muscle imbalances, or injury. A sample training session for an experienced and technically competent adolescent is provided in table 4.2.

Table 4.2 Sample Training Session for a Technically Competent Adolescent With 6 Years of Training Experience

Phase	Exercise	Description	Volume (sets × reps)	Intensity (% 1RM)	Rest (min)
Physical Preparation	Foam rolling	Child gently rolls specific body parts over the top of the foam roller, paying particular focus to areas of muscle tightness or soreness.	2 × 10 (each side)	N/A	1
	Mini-band walks	Child steps laterally with mini band positioned just above the knee or around the ankles.	2 × 10 (each side)	N/A	1
	Glute bridges	Laying on their backs with knees raised and feet in contact with the floor, the children squeeze their glutes to extend their hips towards the ceiling.	2 × 10 (each side)	N/A	1
	Single-leg hop and hold		2 × 4 (each leg)	N/A	1
Main	30 cm (11.8 inches) drop jumps		4 × 3	Bodyweight	1-2
	Power clean		4 × 2	85	2-3
	Back Squat		4 × 5	85	2-3
	Jump Squat		4 × 4	30	2-3

One Size Does Not Fit All: The Need for Flexible Programming

Table 4.2 outlines an approach a practitioner might take to develop neuromuscular power in an adolescent who has engaged in formalized training during childhood. However, this plan may not be appropriate for an athlete who has not achieved an adequate training age and does not possess the technical competency necessary to engage in advanced training strategies. In this situation, the practitioner should still base the training prescription on technical competency; however, the pedagogy involved in coaching more basic training methods (fundamental motor skills) to older youth will likely differ from those used for younger children. Additionally, while possibly possessing greater levels of muscular strength, untrained adolescents lack flexibility or have muscle imbalances that should be addressed in the early stages of the program before attempting to specifically develop neuromuscular power. Conversely, if you're coaching a naturally gifted and highly athletic child, he or she should be allowed to progress to more advanced training strategies or increased intensities while being careful not to sacrifice technical competency. These scenarios underscore the need for practitioners to take a flexible and individualized approach to training youth.

TRAINING OLDER ADULTS

The ability of older (≥65 years) adults to produce power is thought to be vital for retaining neuromuscular function as they age as well as for preventing falls, which can lead to increased morbidity and mortality (3, 26, 76). Retaining neuromuscular function is important for a variety of reasons, including the ability to perform the activities of daily living and preserve muscle mass, which is essential for maintaining a healthy body composition and weight (49, 58, 67). Just like youth, older adults best develop neuromuscular power through resistance training, including explosive, or ballistic, movements and heavily loaded movements. However, older adults should keep physical limitations in mind and perform this type of training only after developing a strength base (63). Therefore, practitioners who choose to incorporate power training into the resistance exercise programs of older adults should conduct a thorough needs analysis and medical history. They should also hold a recognized strength and conditioning qualification, ideally one specific to the older population, and understand the expected physiological and biomechanical responses and adaptations in older adults.

Neuromuscular Decline With Aging

To understand the potential training adaptations to a strength and power training program in the older population, it is necessary to first be familiar with typical decline in physiological functioning of the muscular, neural, and skeletal systems. One of the most evident changes in the aging body is muscular atrophy, or the loss of muscle mass. Sarcopenia is the loss of skeletal muscle mass, quality, and strength associated with aging (19, 38, 64). Much of this total muscle mass loss is caused by disproportionate losses of the faster-contracting Type II muscle fibers (38, 75), likely the result of a reduction in high-force and rapid, explosive activities (19). In conjunction with the Type II muscle fiber atrophy, the related motor neurons also decline in function, firing at a lower rate in their range (81, 82). In addition, the motor unit (a group of muscle fibers and the motor neuron that controls them) remodels, resulting in denervation of the Type II muscle fibers and reinnervation by the neurons associated with the slower-contracting Type I muscle fibers (81, 82). Other changes brought on with age include decreased amounts of myelin covering the motor neuron and reduced transmission of the neural signal to the muscle cells (33, 34, 81). Combined, these alterations reduce force production and contraction speed, thereby reducing power production in aging muscle.

Connective tissue that forms the joints and other connections between the muscles and bones loses some of its elasticity, and increases in stiffness beyond what is optimal for the translation of force from the muscle to the tendon (1). The ability of the tendon to absorb muscle force and store it as potential energy is critical to the functioning of the stretch-shortening cycle (SSC). Therefore, reduced storage of elastic energy results in a reduction in force and power production (1). Between the ages of 30 and 50, strength and power decline gradually. The greatest decline in strength and power occurs after the age of 60, with power showing a more rapid decline than strength. For example, between ages 60 and 65 and 80 and 85, strength levels decline on average about 1% or more per year, which seems minimal, but in 20 years could be as high as 25%-30% (64, 75). Loss of power is more on the magnitude of 3% per year during this same age range, so functional losses are much more visible in the same 20-year period (8, 63, 75).

Trainability of Power in the Older Population

Numerous investigations have used a variety of power training modalities and programming in older populations (80). The most common modalities have been hydraulic or pneumatic resistance exercise machines and free weights (16, 24, 58, 61, 67), and the most common tests involved a countermovement jump or exercises performed with the intent to move rapidly (e.g., double-leg press in a pneumatic or hydraulic machine) (10, 49). Because of the previously mentioned neural decline with aging, machine exercises may be easier for novice lifters to learn because the movements are less complex and are generally restricted to one plane of movement, which should improve safety. In addition, hydraulic or pneumatic resistance is accommodating, and adjusts to the lifter's level of effort. Performance in these exercises is less limited by the load than with free weights, which should also increase safety. However, more highly trained lifters should be able to use free weights effectively. Across any age, the relationship between muscular strength and neuromuscular power is the same, and stronger people have greater capacity to produce power (13). Thus, the benefits of power training in older populations are better realized after establishing a strength base. The other primary component of power—movement speed—can be addressed successfully in a power training program for older adults (20, 24, 54, 73). While the magnitude of improvement in power is more modest than in a young person, positive functional adaptations are nonetheless possible and studies have trained power in older adults with varying levels of success (32, 54, 59, 61, 68, 72).

More specifically, power training can be approached in two ways. The most common is to perform high-speed explosive movements (29, 56, 62), while the other method is to perform movements with the intent to move quickly (4, 49), which may or may not be possible based on the load. Each approach has pros and cons. Performing exercises explosively requires applying more braking force in order to slow the movement before reaching the end of the range of motion. The exception is if the exercise allows a full range of motion at top speed, such as a jump squat, leg-press throw, or bench press throw because the body breaks contact with the ground (jump squat) or with the weight (leg-press throw or bench press throw). While a jump squat does not require specialized equipment (although performing it in a power rack would be safer), and most free-weight leg-press machines can accommodate explosive repetitions, a bench press throw requires the use of a Smith machine for safety purposes. Because of the previously mentioned losses in muscle mass, motor neuron function, and elasticity in the connective tissues, older lifters are even more affected by the higher forces seen in explosive power exercises. This has implications for injury risk, so the emphasis must first be on ensuring that a strength base is present and that exercise technique is flawless. Pneumatic or hydraulic machine exercises have the advantage that movements can be performed with the intent to move fast but without the ballistic characteristics at the end of the joint's range of motion. This is because accommodating resistance only allows for the speed that the lifter can exert, and lifters are mechanically weaker at the ends of the range of motion, so the movement will be slower. A drawback is that many of these exercises take place in a fixed plane of movement and are less likely to mimic normal movements.

Assessing Power in Older Populations

The most common types of equipment used to assess neuromuscular power in older adults include force plates and linear-position transducers (10), pneumatic resistance machines (16, 67), dynamometry (61), and accelerometry (66). Especially when combined with electromyogram (EMG), these measurement devices are fairly sensitive to training-induced changes in power in older adults. Because changes in measures of explosive power, for example, vertical jump performance, are smaller and take longer in older adults compared to younger adults, field tests of jumping performance (e.g., vertical-jump testers, contact mats) may not be sensitive enough to detect these subtle changes. However, aside from research purposes, it may not be as important to monitor actual power output in older adults, who generally are not training for a specific event, as it is to measure improvement in performance of activities of daily living.

Translating the Science Into Program Design

The key concept when designing resistance training programs for older adults that include power exercises or a phase of power development is the needs analysis. Individual differences in training and medical histories will heavily influence not only exercise selection but also the periodization of the training (set and rep scheme) as well. Older adults should be cleared by a physician for participation in an exercise program and should not have serious orthopedic or cardiorespiratory conditions or be on medications that may interfere with their ability to exert themselves physically (60). A secondary concept when designing resistance training programs for older populations is the amount of recovery, which is generally suggested to be longer regardless of whether the primary program goal is hypertrophy, strength, or power (e.g., 72 hours instead of 48 hours between sessions). However, no studies have specifically examined physical performance and adaptations after different recovery intervals between workouts in older adults.

After the assessment of the older adult has been completed and, where necessary, a medical clearance has been provided, exercises can be selected. For power training, the most common and effective explosive exercises involve multiple joints and muscles and include machine exercises as well as free-weight exercises such as jump squats and leg-press throws. Practitioners need to keep in mind that developing a strength base for each of these exercises is necessary before attempting to perform them in a ballistic or explosive fashion. Incorporating a variety of exercises into a periodized program is the most beneficial for well-rounded physical development, but an older adult may need more time to learn each exercise thoroughly and be able to perform each with proper technique because of the motor unit recruitment changes that occur with aging (81, 82). Therefore, it may be best not to rotate exercises too frequently within the program, especially for a novice lifter.

Once the exercises have been chosen, incorporating them into a periodized program is the next step (chapter 3). Some exercises may not be performed in a particular program phase because they are not the best choice for the set and rep scheme in that phase (e.g., should avoid isolation exercises for heavier loading periods), so it is important to think through which exercises will be performed during each primary training goal (e.g., hypertrophy, strength, power). For the novice older lifter, the focus of each phase is more singular. Muscle development (hypertrophy) should be the initial focus, followed by strength development, and then followed by power development (see table 4.3). A more highly trained older adult may spend less time on strength development if the primary training goal is power, or more quickly progress through a mix of exercise styles in a particular phase (see table 4.4).

One aspect that strength and conditioning professionals may struggle with is how best to load the exercise when training for power with older adults. Unfortunately, this issue is the most confusing because power can be increased in older people using loads of 20%-80% of maximum (16, 17, 24, 68). Ideally, a variety of loads will be used, but load determination is influenced by both the exercise selection and the ultimate goal of training (see chapter 3). Some researchers have shown that balance and gait speed are more positively affected by loads in the lower end of the training range (body weight to about 40% of maximum), while getting up out of a chair or climbing steps are more positively affected by loads of 50%-80% of maximum (14, 68). Phases of a program that use these varying loads can also vary in length. In more highly trained older adults, a short phase (2 weeks) may effectively be employed, while a more frail novice lifter may need 8 weeks to make significant improvements (see tables 4.3 and 4.4).

Otherwise, program design for older adults is not that dissimilar to a design for a younger adult, with the exception of a slower overall progression. Loads are relative to the person's own strength levels, and programming should be goal driven, with variety and adequate recovery (see figure 4.2).

Table 4.3 Sample Free-Weight Power Training Program for a Novice Older Adult Lifter

	DAY 1									
Exercise	Week 1-2	Week 3-5	Week 6-8	Week 9-11	Week 12 (recovery)	Week 13-15	Week 16-18	Week 19-21	Week 22-24	Week 25 (recovery)
Back Squat*	1 × 10-12 (50-55%)	2 × 10 (60-65%)	3 × 8 (70-75%)	3 × 6 (80%)	1 × 10 (60%)	3 × 12 (60%)	3 × 10 (65%)	3 × 8 (75%)	3 × 6 (80%)	1 × 10 (60%)
Clean Pull or Power Clean from Blocks	1 × 6 (50-55%)	2 × 6 (60-65%)	3 × 5 (70-75%)	3 × 5 (80%)	1 × 6 (60%)	3 × 6 (60%)	3 × 6 (65%)	3 × 5 (75%)	3 × 5 (80%)	1 × 6 (60%)
Push-ups or Band Push-ups*	1 × 10-12	2 × 10	2 × 8	2 × 6	1 × 10	2 × 12	2 × 10	2 × 8	2 × 6	1 × 10
Dumbbell Push Press	1 × 10-12 (50-55%)	2 × 10 (60-65%)	2 × 8 (70-75%)	2 × 6 (80%)	1 × 10 (60%)	2 × 12 (60%)	2 × 10 (65%)	2 × 8 (75%)	2 × 6 (80%)	1 × 10 (60%)
Bench Pull	1 × 10-12 (50-55%)	2 × 10 (60-65%)	2 × 8 (70-75%)	2 × 6 (80%)	1 × 10 (60%)	2 × 12 (60%)	2 × 10 (65%)	2 × 8 (75%)	2 × 6 (80%)	1 × 10 (60%)
	DAY 2									
Back Squat*	1 × 10-12 (50-55%)	2 × 10 (60-65%)	3 × 8 (70-75%)	3 × 6 (80%)	1 × 10 (60%)					1 × 10 (60%)
Band Standing Rows	1 × 10-12 (50-55%)	2 × 10 (60-65%)	3 × 8 (70-75%)	3 × 6 (80%)	1 × 10 (60%)	2 × 12 (60%)	2 × 10 (65%)	2 × 8 (75%)	2 × 6 (80%)	1 × 10 (60%)
Push-ups or Band Push-ups**	1 × 10-12	2 × 10	2 × 8	2 × 6	1 × 10					1 × 10
Dumbbell Push Press	1 × 10-12 (50-55%)	2 × 10 (60-65%)	2 × 8 (70-75%)	2 × 6 (80%)	1 × 10 (60%)	2 × 12 (60%)	2 × 10 (65%)	2 × 8 (75%)	2 × 6 (80%)	1 × 10 (60%)
Bench Pull	1 × 10-12 (50-55%)	2 × 10 (60-65%)	2 × 8 (70-75%)	2 × 6 (80%)	1 × 10 (60%)	2 × 12 (60%)	2 × 10 (65%)	2 × 8 (75%)	2 × 6 (80%)	1 × 10 (60%)
Jump Squats						3 × 4 (30%)	3 × 5 (35%)	3 × 5 (40%)	3 × 4 (45%)	
Squat Jumps						3 × 4 (30%)	3 × 5 (35%)	3 × 5 (40%)	3 × 4 (45%)	
Bench Press						2 × 12 (60%)	2 × 10 (65%)	2 × 8 (75%)	2 × 6 (80%)	1 × 10 (60%)

*Can be replaced with leg press if required

**Can be performed as assisted push-ups or band push-ups depending on capability of the person.

Table 4.4 Sample Free-Weight Power Training Program for an Experienced Older Adult Lifter

Exercise	Week 1-2	Week 3-5	Week 6-8	Week 9-11	Week 12 (recovery)	Week 13-15	Week 16-18	Week 19-21	Week 22-24	Week 25 (recovery)
DAY 1										
Back Squat*	2 × 10-12 (60-65%)	3 × 10 (65-70%)	3 × 8 (75-80%)	3 × 6 (80-85%)	1 × 10 (65%)	3 × 12 (60%)	3 × 10 (65%)	3 × 8 (75%)	3 × 6 (80%)	1 × 10 (65%)
Clean Pull	2 × 6 (60-65%)	3 × 6 (65-70%)	3 × 5 (75-80%)	3 × 5 (85%)	1 × 6 (65%)	3 × 6 (60%)	3 × 6 (65%)	3 × 5 (75%)	3 × 5 (80%)	1 × 6 (65%)
Bench Press	2 × 10-12 (60-65%)	3 × 10 (65-70%)	2 × 8 (75-80%)	2 × 6 (80-85%)	1 × 10 (65%)	2 × 12 (60%)	2 × 10 (65%)	2 × 8 (75%)	2 × 6 (80%)	1 × 10 (65%)
Dumbbell Push Press	2 × 8-10 (60-65%)	3 × 8 (65-70%)	2 × 6 (75-80%)	2 × 5 (85%)	1 × 10 (65%)	2 × 10 (65%)	2 × 8 (70%)	2 × 6 (75%)	2 × 5 (80%)	1 × 10 (65%)
Bench Pull	2 × 10-12 (60-65%)	3 × 10 (65-70%)	2 × 8 (75-80%)	2 × 5 (85%)	1 × 10 (65%)	2 × 10 (65%)	2 × 8 (70%)	2 × 6 (75%)	2 × 6 (80%)	1 ×10 (65%)
DAY 2										
Back Squat*	2 × 10-12 (60-65%)	3 × 10 (65-70%)	3 × 8 (75-80%)	3 × 5 (85%)						
Clean Pull	2 × 6 (60-65%)	3 × 6 (65-70%)	3 × 6 (75-80%)	3 × 5 (85%)		2 × 6 (60%)	2 × 6 (65%)	2 × 5 (75%)	2 × 5 (80%)	
Bench Press	2 × 10-12 (60-65%)	3 ×10 (65-70%)	2 × 8 (75-80%)	2 × 6 (80-85%)	1 × 10 (65%)					1 × 10 (65%)
Dumbbell Push Press	2 × 8-10 (60-65%)	3 × 8 (65-70%)	2 × 6 (75-80%)	2 × 5 (85%)	1 × 10 (65%)	2 × 12 (60%)	2 × 10 (65%)	2 × 8 (75%)	2 × 6 (80%)	1 × 10 (65%)
Bench Pull	2 × 10-12 (60-65%)	3 × 10 (65-70%)	2 × 6 (75-80%)	2 × 5 (85%)	1 × 10 (65%)	2 × 12 (60%)	2 × 10 (65%)	2 × 8 (75%)	2 × 6 (80%)	1 × 10 (65%)
Jump Squats						3 × 6 (30%)	3 × 6 (40%)	3 × 4 (50%)	3 × 5 (50%)	
Squat Jumps						3 × 6 (30%)	3 × 6 (40%)	3 × 4 (50%)	3 × 5 (50%)	
Band Standing Row					1 × 10 (65%)	2 × 12 (60%)	2 × 10 (65%)	2 × 8 (75%)	2 × 6 (80%)	1 × 10 (65%)

*Can be replaced with leg press if required

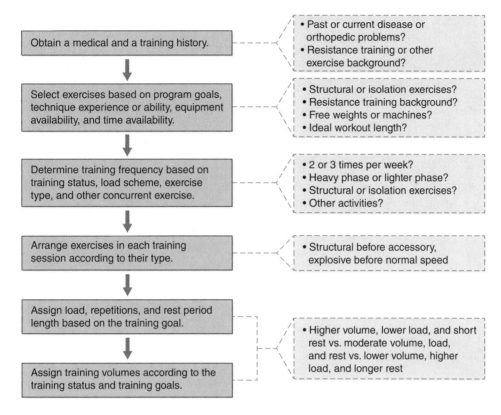

Figure 4.2 Steps for constructing a periodized program for an older adult.

CONCLUSION

When developing neuromuscular power in youth, practitioners should consider the following key points:

▶ Both children and adolescents will naturally increase neuromuscular power as a result of growth and maturation.

▶ All youth can make worthwhile gains in neuromuscular power when exposed to developmentally appropriate training programs.

▶ While enhancing neuromuscular power might be the ultimate aim of a youth-based strength and conditioning program, practitioners should first look to develop motor skill competency and requisite levels of muscular strength.

▶ Irrespective of whether the training program attempts to develop motor skills, muscular strength, or indeed neuromuscular power, progression should be based on a combination of technical competency, training age, and biological and psychosocial maturation.

▶ Practitioners must be flexible in programming to ensure that the training prescribed meets individual needs.

When a primary training goal is to develop neuromuscular power in an older adult, practitioners should consider the following key points:

▶ Neuromuscular power is a function of both peak strength levels and the ability to perform a movement rapidly.

▶ All older adults have the capacity to improve their neuromuscular power somewhat with well-designed and well-implemented training programs, but the degree to which this occurs depends on their individual physical limitations and medical history.

▶ Training for neuromuscular power should be performed only after an older adult has established a strength base and can perform movements with proper technique both under load and at a rapid speed.

PART II

Exercises for Power Development

CHAPTER 5

Upper Body Power Exercises

Disa L. Hatfield, PhD, CSCS,*D

Upper body power is critical in sports involving over- or underhand throwing, hitting, combat, or propulsion. The physiology and physics of power development of the upper body are the same as that of the lower body. However, upper body power training presents unique training considerations. Variance in recommendations for training intensity based on sex, experience, and sport can make programming for developing upper body power challenging. In addition, the research literature has not adequately addressed many commonly debated issues, such as programming rotational exercises versus isometric exercises to improve abdominal strength. The purpose of this chapter is to address performance aids, training devices, and testing devices that are specific to upper body power training and to provide techniques, instructions, and exercise variations for upper body power exercises.

SPECIAL AIDS FOR UPPER BODY POWER TRAINING

Coaches and athletes are always seeking training devices or aids that will promote athletic performance. Aside from dietary and supplemental ergogenic aids, a variety of products can enhance power training and performance.

Power Training Aids

Medicine balls are a popular training device for use in plyometric training. Medicine balls have evolved over the past 10 years. They now include variations with handles, ropes, and nonrebounding capabilities (soft-toss balls). They come in a variety of sizes and weights. They are widely available at retail stores and through fitness equipment manufacturers and are cost effective compared to other resistance training modalities. Many of the exercises described in this chapter use a medicine ball, which should be the minimum equipment required for upper body power training.

Some powerlifting training approaches include resistance bands in their bench press training (see figure 5.4) to increase rate of force development (RFD). Resistance bands enhance the eccentric loading of an exercise, leading to maximized power output during the concentric phase (5, 17, 22). In addition, proponents of this training method suggest it may be beneficial in decelerating bar speed (22). However, research concerning the effectiveness of using bands to increase strength is conflicting and fraught with potential validity issues (5, 8, 21, 22, 32). To date, only one study has measured upper body power after training with bands, and it reported no significant differences between the results of resistance band training and seven weeks of free-weight bench press training (17). One potential drawback to using resistance bands during traditional free-weight training is that intensity of the load is not easily characterized because of individual differences in bar path trajectory and length with and without bands. While the current literature is too sparse to recommend the addition of resistance band training as a necessary component of power training, it can be considered a novel addition to training that has both potential benefits and limitations. These modalities are discussed in more detail in chapter 8.

Acute Performance Aids

Only a small body of literature looks at specialized aids that will improve upper body power production in an acute setting, such as an individual training session. One study suggests that wearing a specially fitted mouth guard during bench press throwing increases power production in both men and women (13). However, athletic performance parameters such as throwing velocity were not assessed, and this finding has not been replicated in other resistance training studies.

The use of compression garments as an acute athletic performance aid is not fully understood. Some evidence suggests that compression garments may aid in recovery after a strenuous resistance training session, but the information specific to performance (18, 19, 25) is limited. Only one current study has addressed sport-specific upper body power or anaerobic performance (19). The authors concluded that a compression garment did improve accuracy in both athletes, but did not affect golf swing velocity or throwing velocity. Among other possibilities, this may suggest that the proprioceptive feedback a compression garment offers may be useful in an acute performance setting in which power and accuracy are both important.

Despite little research in this area, compression garments for upper body athletic performance are popular in certain athletic populations, particularly powerlifters. Powerlifters frequently wear garments called bench shirts to enhance their bench press performance. These shirts are made of a variety of materials, from single-ply polyester to multi-ply denim. They are tight fitting and designed to offer aid during the concentric portion of the exercise because of the proposed benefit of greater stored energy during the eccentric portion of the exercise. These shirts have led to the development of the Sling Shot used by recreational lifters. The Sling Shot is an elastic band that is worn across the chest while benching. Like a bench press shirt, theoretically, it stores potential energy as it is stretched on the eccentric portion of the exercise, allowing for a more powerful concentric muscle action.

Bar Speed and Power Measuring Devices to Monitor Training Progress

Independent of athletic performance, a variety of methods are available for monitoring the progress of upper body power training. Commonly used field tests include a simple medicine ball throw for distance, such as a chest pass (see chapter 2). While this method is certainly inexpensive and easy to administer, little normative data is available that can be used for comparing athletes to their like population (16).

Several commercially available devices can measure power and velocity during bar, medicine ball, and body-weight exercises. These devices use either tensiometry, to measure bar speed, or accelerometry, to quantify velocity. While the literature has validated these devices, they can be costly, and like field tests, normative data does not exist for a wide variety of populations (11, 16). Aside from testing, anecdotal evidence suggests that coaches and athletes use some of these devices during training to monitor power and velocity in acute sessions. Athletes typically try to remain within a certain percentage of their maximum power output, and thus receive instant feedback that motivates them to maintain a high power output on each repetition or throw. While kinematic software analysis has been shown to be effective in teaching complex movements, programming based on power output and bar or ball velocity has not been studied (30). The use of velocity-based training (VBT) is discussed in more detail in chapter 8.

UPPER BODY POWER TRAINING CONSIDERATIONS

There are multiple factors to consider when training to enhance upper body power. For instance, production of upper body power happens rarely without concomitant movement from the lower body. Optimizing the transfer of force and power production from lower body movements can enhance upper body power output (referred to as transfer of momentum). In addition, the prescription of acute resistance program variables when training for power, such as intensity, are not as well-defined in evidence-based research as it is for other performance outcomes such as strength.

Transfer of Momentum

Ballistic exercises, in which deceleration of the bar or person is negated, are necessary in upper body power training. Deceleration is needed in exercises such as the bench press, when the bar must slow at the end of a bench press motion so it does not leave the athlete's hands. However, a great amount of eccentric muscle action is necessary to slow the momentum, which can cause injury. In addition, the agonist muscle is not concentrically active through the whole range of motion (ROM). Momentum is the tendency of an object to continue moving and is defined as mass multiplied by velocity. To overcome the deceleration phenomenon, it is necessary to either transfer the momentum to another object or continue to accelerate and allow the bar to leave the athlete's hands, such as in a bench press throw (29). Resistance bands decrease the need for eccentric deceleration by increasing the external resistance through the concentric ROM and allow the muscle to continue to work concentrically through a greater ROM (17, 22).

Multiple studies suggest that upper body power has a significant relationship to lower body power, similar to the relationship it has with dynamic core strength (7, 9, 10). In an acute setting, throwing distance, velocity, and peak power output of the upper body are all significantly increased when lower limbs are used in the movement (7, 9, 10). Motions like throwing a shot put, shooting a basketball, or throwing a punch require a ground-up sequence of activation in which momentum passes from the lower body to torso, torso to shoulder, shoulder to elbow, elbow to wrist and fingers, and finally to the implement (29). Thus, lower body and torso power movements and exercises that transfer momentum through the upper body should be included in acute training sessions and longer-term training programs.

Intensity

Research indicates that the intensity of upper body power training may depend on sex, sport, arm length, and training experience (1, 2, 4). For instance, research indicates that trained athletes produce maximal power at a lower percentage of their 1RM in comparison to the untrained (2, 4). This training adaptation is important because it indicates the ability of trained people to synchronously recruit motor units and shift the force–velocity curve up. In basic terms, trained people are more explosive and require less initial resistance to recruit fast-twitch fibers.

The literature reports that maximal power outputs during a bench press throw in various athletic populations lies between 15% and 60% of 1RM (1, 3, 6, 26, 29). Athletes should strive to perform weighted upper body power exercises at an intensity that produce the highest power. Bar speed measuring devices, as described earlier in this chapter, allow for easy monitoring of power during an exercise like a bench press throw. If these devices are not available, choose loads of 30%-60%. At least one study reports that while upper body peak power occurred at 30% of 1RM in the sample population, there were no significant differences between power at 30%, 40%, or 50% of 1RM (6). In addition, the load that produced peak power in the upper body was different from the load that produced peak power in the lower body. Because of the many factors that influence the load at which peak power occurs, monitoring power during training may be essential for an individualized training prescription.

Regardless, few field-friendly methods of monitoring speed and power while performing upper body power exercises like medicine ball throws and plyometric drills exist. Despite a lack of peer-reviewed recommendations of loading intensity for medicine ball drills, plyometric and medicine ball training have both been shown to improve athletic performance parameters, such as throwing and hitting velocity (9,

16). As such, plyometric and medicine ball training should be thought of as essential to upper body power training because both work to enhance the stretch-shortening cycle (SSC), thus increasing explosive ability and power over time.

Rotator Cuff Mechanics

The muscles of the shoulder joint serve several purposes during power movements, including dynamic stabilization of the joint, force generation, and eccentric deceleration toward the end of full ROM (20, 23, 29). Unlike other joints, the glenohumeral joint is largely unstable because only a small portion of it articulates with the glenoid fossa, and subsequently the purpose of the surrounding musculature is mainly to provide stabilization, not to produce power. The unique functions of these muscles and anatomy of the joint result in a high rate of strain, impingement, and tendinitis of the structures surrounding the shoulder joint (20). Muscular imbalance caused by repetitive motion and overuse is a factor in these injuries (23). Yet despite the incidence of shoulder injury, little research has been conducted concerning strength and conditioning programming of volume, exercise technique, and exercise adaptations that may help reduce the risk of injury in athletes (23). The research that does exist is highly specialized and often uses clinical equipment such as isokinetic machines that are not widely available (16). Probably the most common generalized advice for training rotator cuff mechanics is to address muscular imbalances that may lead to injury (12, 23).

For the purposes of this chapter, coaches and athletes should consider the following:

▶ Despite the lower load of many power exercises, upper body power exercises that contain an enhanced eccentric portion should be classified as high intensity. Partner-assisted loading, rebounding, and resistance band exercises will increase the eccentric loading of the shoulder joint and should be performed in lower volumes. While resistance bands also offer increased resistance at the top end of an exercise, which aids in deceleration of movement, they also increase the eccentric force, which may increase injury potential. The effects of acute and chronic training with these devices on shoulder mechanics and movement has not been addressed.

▶ Release exercises such as the bench press throw and medicine ball exercises can reduce, but not fully negate, the need for deceleration.

▶ No power exercises exist for the rhomboids and latissimus dorsi, which primarily function to stabilize the joint. If an athlete's regular sports training involves repetitive external rotation or pushing motions, muscular imbalances between the anterior and posterior upper body may be exacerbated. While some power exercises use shoulder muscles that are involved in internal and external rotation, very few power exercises work the rear deltoids, rhomboids, and latissimus dorsi. When programming upper body power exercises, equalize the volume for muscle groups that push and pull, or address the volume inequalities in the athletes' traditional strength training routine to prevent muscular imbalances that can lead to rotator cuff injuries (23).

Rotational Exercises

Current literature suggests that isometric core strength is related to injury prevention and athletic performance (14, 24, 27, 28). This, along with concerns that dynamic abdominal exercise exacerbates low back pain, has led to programming solely isometric core exercises such as a plank to improve abdominal strength (27). However, research addressing the role of the trunk muscles in sport performance suggests that dynamic training of the lateral core musculature (e.g., obliques) allows for effective transfer of forces from the lower body and increases power development of the upper body (15, 31). While performance research suggests that athletes should train the movements they will perform in their sport, practitioners should also individually assess lower back injury history and training status and then choose exercises accordingly. In addition, it may be prudent to take into consideration the sport-specific pattern of momentum transfer. For instance, lower limb strength deficits have been reported to disrupt the kinetic chain and contribute to impingement syndrome in the shoulder (20, 23).

UPPER BODY POWER EXERCISES

Choosing exercises to include in a program to train upper body power is dependent on many factors. Some of the considerations are loading, athlete training experience, and type of movement. To better facilitate these choices, exercises described in this chapter are categorized as ballistic, variable resistance (plyometric), or Olympic. Ballistic exercises are traditionally defined as those in which resistive force leaves the athlete's hands or the athlete leaves the ground, negating the need for deceleration during the concentric muscle action (such as a bench press throw). Variable-resistance exercises, such as those done with a resistance band, are included in this category because of the commonality of enhanced eccentric loading they share with ballistic exercises. Plyometric exercises are often ballistic in nature as well, but typically use a medicine ball. For instance, exercises such as bounding or depth jumps are ballistic (the athlete leaves the ground and the concentric portion is not decelerated). However, plyometric exercises also seek to enhance the SSC with an enhanced eccentric component. Olympic lift progression exercises are variations or techniques used as part of the main Olympic lifts (see chapter 7).

Within these categories, exercises are further characterized into novice, intermediate, or advanced levels. Novice exercises use a relatively simple movement patterns and low intensity. Intermediate-level exercises use either a more complex movement pattern or the intensity of the exercise is increased because of an enhanced eccentric portion. Advanced exercises use both a complex movement pattern and a heavier eccentric loading pattern.

BALLISTIC AND VARIABLE-RESISTANCE EXERCISES

JUMP PUSH-UP

Level: Novice

Action

1. Start at the top of a push-up with the head in a neutral position and the arms extended (figure 5.1a).

2. Perform a standard push-up with a full ROM (figure 5.1b), while explosively extending the arms so the hands leave the ground and land in the same place (figure 5.1c).

3. Begin the next repetition immediately after landing.

Variations

See band and depth-drop push-up.

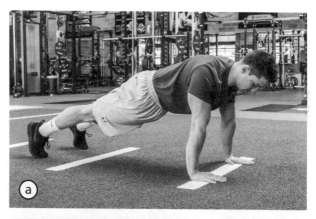

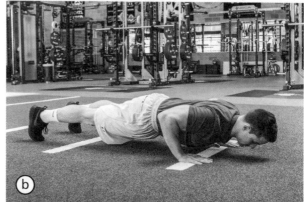

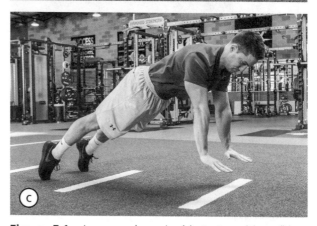

Figure 5.1 Jump push-up in (a) start position, (b) at end of countermovement, and (c) after ballistic concentric action.

BAND PUSH-UP

A band or tubing offers both resistance during the concentric muscle action and an enhanced eccentric action (as opposed to a weight or dumbbell placed on the athlete's back, which doesn't offer enhanced loading).

Level: Intermediate

Action

1. In push-up position, hold one end of a resistance band or tubing in each hand, with the band or tubing running across the upper back and rear deltoids (figure 5.2a).
2. Perform a standard push-up (figure 5.2b).

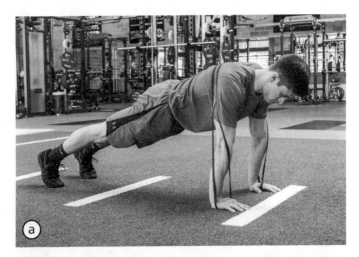

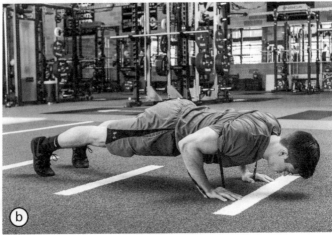

Figure 5.2   Band push-ups in (a) start position and (b) at end of countermovement.

Variations

Increase intensity by leaving the ground, similar to a jump push-up (advanced level).

BENCH PRESS

Level: Intermediate

Action

1. Lie supine on a bench in a five-point body contact position: feet on the floor, head on the bench, buttocks on the bench, and shoulders and upper back in contact with the bench. Optimally, the feet should be as close to the center of the body as possible to facilitate leg drive.

2. Grip the bar with the hands slightly wider than shoulder width.

3. A spotter should help unrack the bar and position it over the center of the chest.

4. Hold the bar with the elbows fully extended above the center of the chest (figure 5.3a).

5. Lower the weight straight down to the center of the chest (between the nipple line and xiphoid process). At the bottom of the movement, the elbows should be slightly tucked toward the body without being perpendicular to the shoulders or close to the body (figure 5.3b).

6. Without bouncing the bar off the chest, extend the elbows and press the weight straight up.

7. Maintain the five-point body contact position during the exercise.

8. The spotter should aid in racking the bar once the exercise is completed.

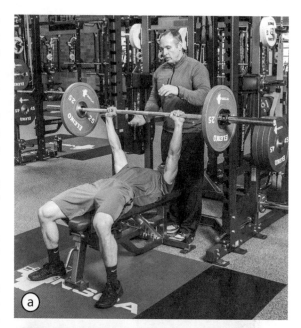

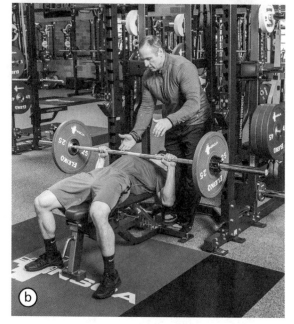

Figure 5.3 Bench press *(a)* start and *(b)* end positions.

BAND BENCH PRESS

Level: Advanced

Action

1. Perform this exercise using the same form as a standard flat barbell bench press (figure 5.3).
2. Loop resistance bands (resistance tubing is not strong enough for this exercise) on both sides of the bar on the inside of the sleeve close to the weights.
3. Attach the other end of the band to a rack (newer models come with hooks on the edge of the platform near the floor) or to a heavy dumbbell placed on the floor. If you use dumbbells, they should be heavy enough that they won't be lifted during the movement. Typically, total dumbbell weight should exceed bar weight.
4. Spotter duties are similar to those for the barbell bench press. However, the added resistance of the bands will increase the tension when the spotter hands off the bar and may also lead to more instability during the handoff. The spotter should release the bar smoothly into the lifter's hands. In addition, the spotter is at added risk because of the potential for the bands to snap or the dumbbells to roll.
5. The band should be as vertical as possible when bar is unracked and in the standard start position (figure 5.4a).
6. The resistance band will offer an enhanced eccentric load and more resistance at the end of the concentric action to help slow the movement velocity. This tension can lead to wavering of the bar if the lifter does not have complete control of the bar and can also lead to a rebound effect at the end of the movement when the band "snaps" the bar back down.
7. Focus on moving the bar explosively through a full ROM but without bouncing the bar off the chest (figure 5.4b).

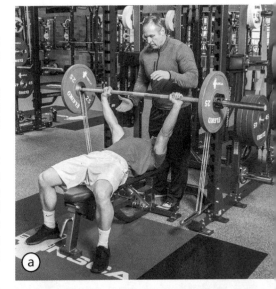

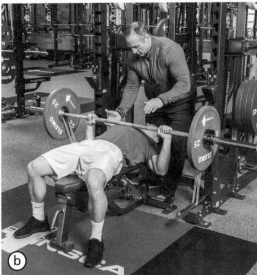

Figure 5.4 Band bench press in (a) start position and (b) at the end of countermovement.

Variations

You can affect the intensity by varying the weight on the bar and the length and thickness of the resistance band. Coaches and athletes should consider this a power movement and therefore choose a load and resistance band that the athlete can move with great velocity.

BENCH PRESS THROW ON SMITH MACHINE

Level: Advanced

Action

1. Most Smith machines come equipped with a safety lock or racks that can be set to just above chest level or both, meaning the bar will not touch the athlete's chest. Set the safety locks at a height that prevents the bar from landing on the lifter if the lifter and spotter both fail to catch the bar.
2. Use a spotter for this exercise.
3. The start position is the same as for a standard flat barbell bench press (figure 5.3). Carefully unrack the weight and hold with arms extended. The spotter helps the lifter unrack the bar. If the lifter rotated his hands during the unrack, the lifter should reposition his hands to the appropriate spot after turning the bar to unlock it from the rack (i.e., re-grip). If this is necessary, the spotter should help stabilize the bar during this process.
4. Begin by flexing the elbows and lowering bar toward the chest.
5. At the bottom of the movement, rapidly extend the elbows and release the bar when the elbows reach full extension.
6. Catch the bar in its downward path, quickly lower it to a self-selected depth, and then begin the next repetition. The spotter should help catch the bar to make sure the athlete has control, and the safety locks should be positioned so that the bar cannot touch the lifter's chest.
7. The spotter should remain diligent during the entire motion to help the athlete catch the bar.

Variations

Devices are available that attach to the bar and automatically catch the bar when it starts to descend after the throw; however, these also negate the optimized eccentric loading of the exercise.

BAND STANDING ROW

Level: Novice

Action

1. Attach a resistance band to a wall hook or wrap the band securely around a stable rack at approximately chest level.
2. Stand with the feet shoulder-width apart and grasp the ends of the band.
3. Start the movement with the arms fully extended and the band held taut, but not stretched (figure 5.5*a*).
4. Fully flex the elbows to perform a rowing movement through a full ROM (figure 5.5*b*), then quickly return to the starting position and begin the next repetition.

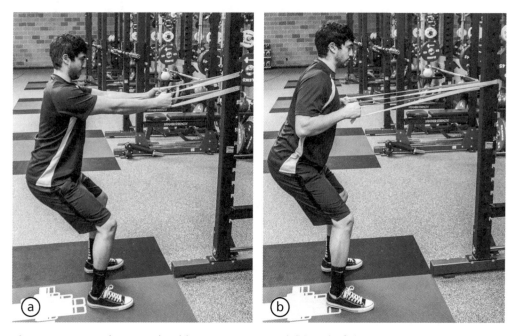

Figure 5.5 Band row at the *(a)* start position and *(b)* end of the countermovement.

Variations

- Intensity depends on the thickness and length of the band used and the distance the athlete stands from the band attachment site.
- This exercise can be varied in the same manner as a barbell or dumbbell row exercise.

SWISS BALL SHOULDER ROLL

Level: Novice

Action

1. Lie prone with arms and legs extended over a Swiss ball. The ball should be large enough that the feet touch the ground in the starting position (figure 5.6a).

2. Carefully flex the knees. Then, extend the legs rapidly while the trunk rolls over the ball.

3. Once the hands reach the floor, flex the elbows for the countermovement (figure 5.6b).

4. Rapidly extend the elbows and roll back to the starting position.

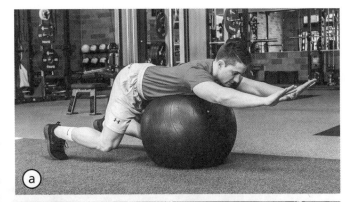

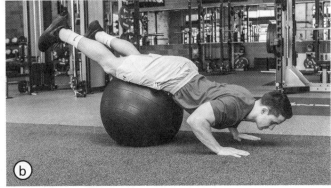

Figure 5.6 Swiss ball shoulder roll in *(a)* start position, and *(b)* at the end of countermovement.

BENCH PULL

Level: Intermediate

Action

1. Lie prone on a bench, gripping the bar with a closed, pronated grip slightly wider than shoulder width (figure 5.7a).
2. The height of the bench should be set so the athlete can hold the bar in a hanging position with the weight off the ground.
3. Lift the bar from the hang position, pulling the bar toward the lower chest with the elbows pointing upward and the head remaining in contact with the bench (figure 5.7b).
4. Pull the bar up until it lightly touches the underside of the bench and then lower it in a controlled fashion to full elbow extension without touching the floor.

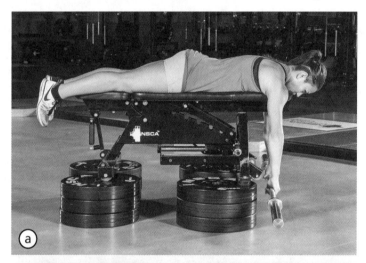

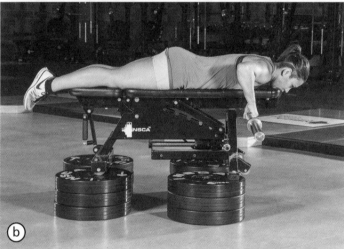

Figure 5.7 Bench pull at the (a) start position and (b) during the lifting motion.

DEPTH-DROP PUSH-UP

Level: Advanced

Action

1. Begin at the bottom of the push-up position with hands on raised platforms (of equal height) that are placed on either side of the shoulders. Generally, the height of the blocks, platforms or sometimes bumper plates used is between two and six inches (5 – 15 cm) (figure 5.8a).

2. Begin the movement by extending the arms.

3. Move the hands off the platform and onto the floor (figure 5.8b).

4. Explosively extend the arms so that the hands leave the ground (figure 5.8c) and land back on the platform.

The platform height varies depending on the intensity desired, experience, and the length of the athlete's arms. Higher platforms will result in greater eccentric loading and are more appropriate for experienced athletes.

Variations

- Begin at the bottom position of the push-up, with hands on top of a medicine ball (in line with the upper chest) and the arms extended.

- Move the hands from the ball to the floor (approximately shoulder-width apart) and perform a push-up to the level of the ball.

- Explosively extend the arms so that the hands leave the ground and land back on the medicine ball.

- Medicine ball height varies depending on intensity desired, experience, and arm length of the athlete.

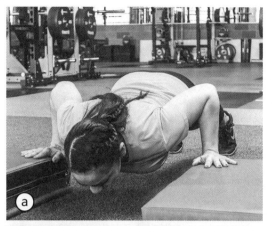

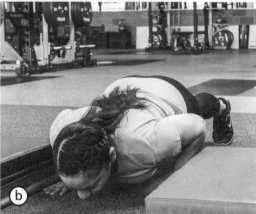

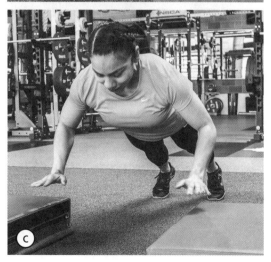

Figure 5.8 Depth-drop push-up in (a) start position, (b) at the end of countermovement, and (c) after the ballistic concentric action.

CHEST PASS

Level: Novice

Action

1. Stand with the feet shoulder-width apart.
2. Hold a medicine ball at the center of the chest (figure 5.9*a*).
3. Perform with a countermovement by flexing the elbows before the throw.
4. Slightly flex the knees and hips to produce a lower body countermovement (figure 5.9*b*).
5. During knee and hip extension, extend the arms and release the ball at full extension (figure 5.9*c*).

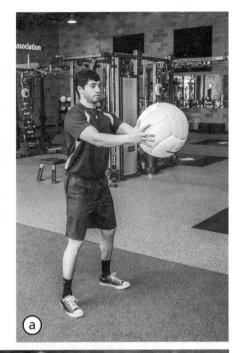

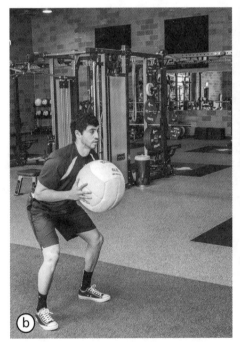

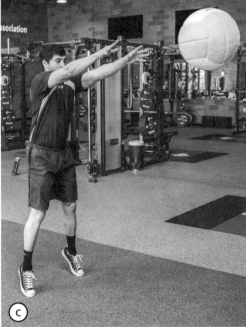

Figure 5.9 Chest pass in *(a)* start position, *(b)* at the end of the countermovement, and *(c)* after the ballistic concentric action.

Variations

- Perform chest passes as quickly as possible with a partner to allow for enhanced eccentric loading and optimization of the SSC.
- For a deltoid exercise, throw the medicine ball straight up into the air from the center of the chest. Ensure no one else is in the immediate area in case the throw goes awry and the athlete must be prepared to catch the ball on the descent.
- To perform the exercise without a partner, throw a larger soft-toss (nonbounce) medicine ball against a wall. These balls diminish the rebound effect.
- Start in the original stance on both feet. As the ball releases, explosively jump forward off one leg and land on the opposite foot as in a forward pass in basketball. This is an intermediate-level exercise (figure 5.9d).
- Perform the exercise using a rebounder, such as a vertically mounted trampoline (intermediate level).

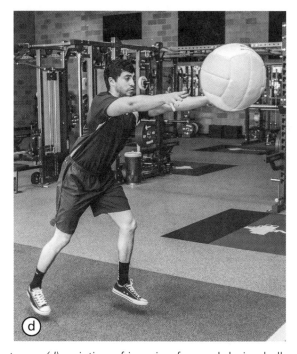

Figure 5.9 Chest pass (d) variation of jumping forward during ball release.

SCOOP TOSS

Level: Novice

Action

1. Stand with the feet shoulder-width apart.
2. Hold a medicine ball at hip level with the arms fully extended (figure 5.10*a*).
3. Perform the countermovement by flexing the hips and knees to approximately a half-squat position (figure 5.10*b*).
4. Concentrically extend the knees and hips while externally rotating at the shoulders to throw the ball up and backward over the head in a rapid and controlled manner (figure 5.10*c*).

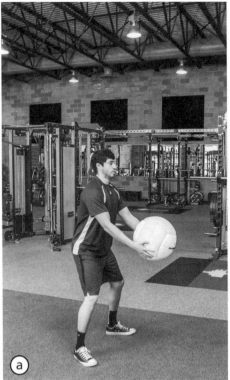

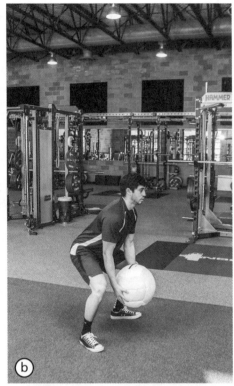

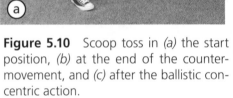

Figure 5.10 Scoop toss in (a) the start position, (b) at the end of the counter-movement, and (c) after the ballistic concentric action.

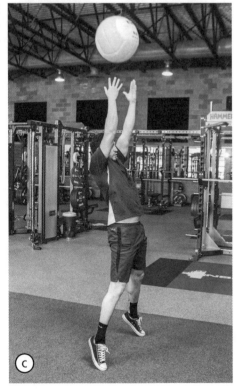

LATERAL TOSS (LOW HOLD AND HIGH HOLD)

Level: Intermediate

Action

1. Stand with the feet shoulder-width apart in an athletic stance (knees and hips slightly flexed).
2. Hold a medicine ball at midtorso level with the arms extended (figure 5.11a).
3. The initial countermovement is a rotation at the waist with concurrent knee and hip flexion and a slight lowering of the medicine ball to about thigh level (low hold) (figure 5.11b).
4. Concentrically extend the knees and hips while rotating the opposite direction to throw the ball laterally and slightly up (figure 5.11c).
5. Repeat set starting from a right rotation and throwing left.

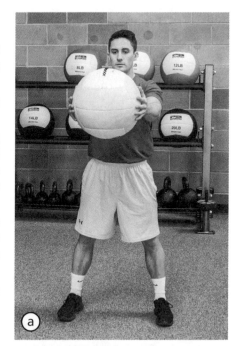

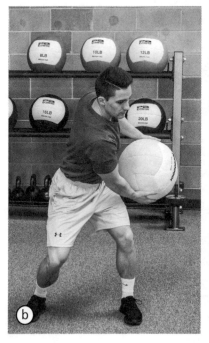
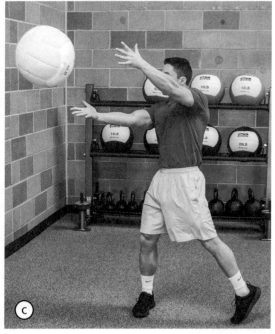

Figure 5.11 Lateral toss (low hold and high hold) at (a) the start position, (b) at the end of the low-hold countermovement, and (c) after the low-hold ballistic concentric action.

Variations

- In the high-hold variation, hold the ball at midtorso and project the ball straight instead of slightly up (figure 5.11*d-e*).
- Pass rapidly with a partner.
- Rebound against a wall using a larger soft-toss ball and a high hold (distance from wall varies based on ability, but generally is 2-3 ft [0.6-1 m]).
- Perform exercise using a rebounder, such as a vertically mounted trampoline.

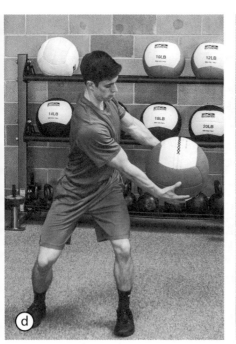 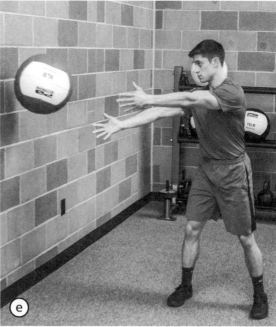

Figure 5.11 Lateral toss high-hold variation *(d)* at the high position at the end of counter-movement, and *(e)* after the high-hold ballistic concentric action.

OVERHEAD THROW

Level: Intermediate

Action

1. Stand with the feet shoulder-width apart.

2. Hold a medicine ball in front of the body with the arms extended (figure 5.12a).

3. Flex the shoulders to lift the ball over and slightly behind the head (figure 5.12b).

4. Keeping the elbows extended, extend the shoulders to throw the ball toward a wall; be sure to release the ball while it is still over the head (figure 5.12c).

5. Aim the ball at a spot on the wall so that when it rebounds the ball returns to the hands that are still positioned overhead.

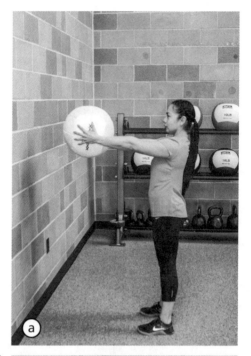

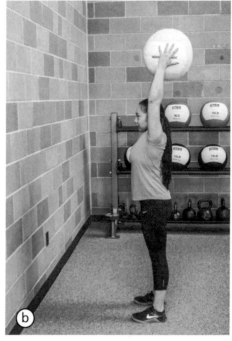

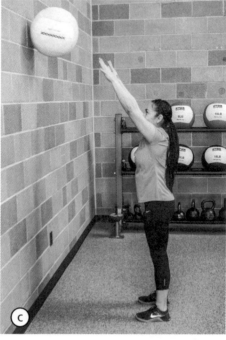

Figure 5.12 Overhead throw at (a) the start position, (b) at the end of the counter-movement, and (c) after the ballistic concentric action.

Variations

- Throw for distance instead of using a wall for the rebound (novice level).
- Instead of releasing the ball overhead, maintain contact with the ball and slam it toward the ground while simultaneously flexing the knees and hips to about a quarter-squat position. This is a novice-level variation, commonly called a medicine ball slam; use a soft-toss ball for minimal rebound.
- For an advanced variation, use a split stance and an explosive forward jump during the overhead throw; maintain awareness of the rebound (figure 5.12d).
- For an intermediate variation, use a rebounder.

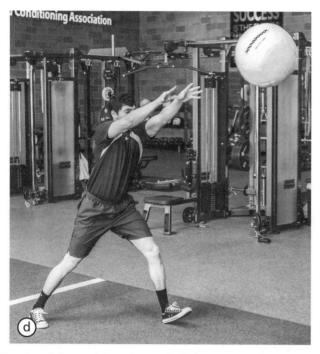

Figure 5.12 Overhead throw (d) at the end of the concentric action of the overhead throw variation.

TWO-HANDED WOOD CHOP THROW

Level: Intermediate

Action

1. Stand with the feet shoulder-width apart.
2. Hold a medicine ball at the center of the chest (figure 5.13a).
3. Similar to a low-hold lateral toss, rotate right at the waist with concurrent knee and hip flexion and lower the medicine ball to about knee level (arms should be fully extended to reach this position); greater knee flexion should occur in the left leg (figure 5.13b).
4. While extending the knees and hips, move the ball in an arc, ending with the ball over the right side of the head (figure 5.13c).
5. Explosively throw the ball toward the ground (figure 5.13d).
6. Repeat the movement but rotate to the left and throw the medicine ball toward the ground on the right side.

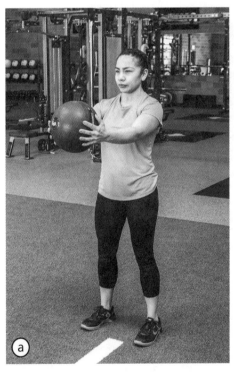 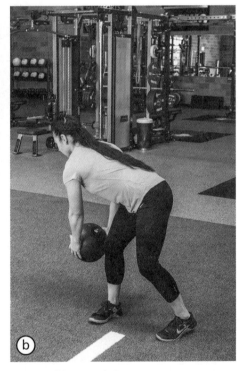

Figure 5.13 Wood chop at (a) the start position, (b) end of the countermovement, (c) end of hip and knee extension just before the ball release, and (d) release of the ball toward the ground.

Variations

- Use a soft-toss ball for limited rebound.
- If using a standard medicine ball, catch the rebound and immediately begin the sequence again (advanced level).
- To negate the initial countermovement and leg actions, start the exercise holding the ball overhead and to the right; the second motion is throwing the ball to the ground in a fashion similar to chopping wood (novice level).
- In all variations, the ball projection can be a forward and diagonal throw with a partner or rebounder or for distance.
- For an advanced variation, athletes can perform this movement using a sledgehammer and a large tractor tire. The sledgehammer replaces the ball, but follows the same motion pathway as it slams onto the large tire lying on its side (but strike the tire slightly off-center so the sledgehammer does not bounce back up to the face). The tractor tire works as a rebound device and also allows for transfer of momentum. Be careful not to hit the sledgehammer too close to the edge of the tire, which can cause the tire bounce up. Also, do not release the handle of the sledgehammer upon striking the tire. The head of a sledgehammer can weigh 1-9 kg (2-20 lb). The weight of the sledgehammer should reflect the abilities of the athlete.

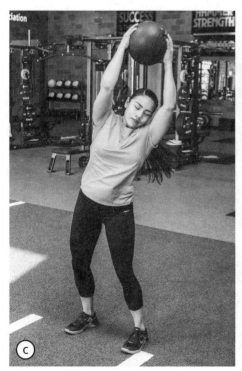

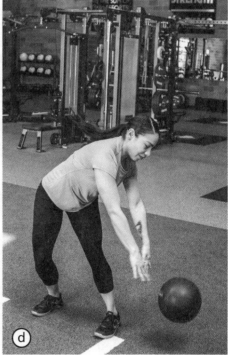

ABDOMINAL CRUNCH BALL TOSS

Level: Advanced

Action

1. Begin in a sit-up position with the knees flexed, the feet flat the ground, and the arms slightly flexed at the elbows. Hold a medicine ball at the center of the chest (figure 5.14a).

2. A partner stands 1-3 feet (0.3-1 m) away ready to catch the ball.

3. Perform a standard abdominal crunch and extend the arms at the elbows to explosively throw the ball toward the partner (see figure 5.14b).

4. As the athlete is in the process of lowering the upper body back to the starting position, the partner performs a chest pass (figure 5.14c) to toss the medicine ball back to the athlete who catches it during the lowering movement. The repetition ends with the athlete and the ball in the starting position (figure 5.14a).

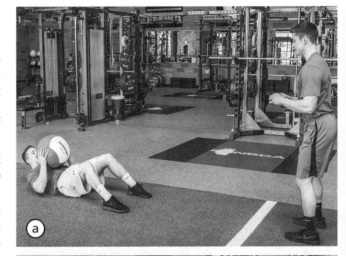

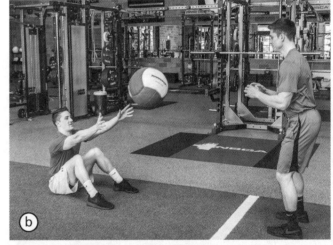

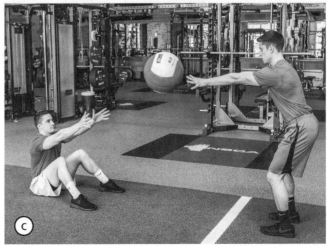

Figure 5.14 Abdominal crunch ball toss at (a) the start position, (b) at the end of the concentric action just after the ball release, and (c) after the partner performed the chest pass.

Variations

With two partners standing to the right and left, perform a slight rotation during the crunch movement and toss the ball to the partner on the right, receive the ball from the partner, and repeat the movement to the left (figure 5.14*d*).

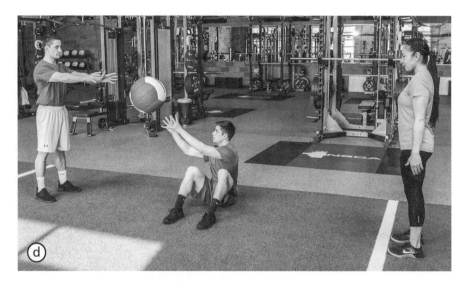

Figure 5.14   Abdominal crunch ball toss *(d)* during the variation of ball release with torso twist to a partner standing on each side.

BALL DROP

Level: Advanced

Action

1. Begin by lying with the back flat on the ground and a partner standing on a box placed near the head.

2. Fully extend the arms toward the sky or ceiling at shoulder level (not above the face) (figure 5.15a).

3. The partner holds the medicine ball and drops it straight into the athlete's hands.

4. After catching the ball, immediately flex at the elbows, bringing the ball to chest level (figure 5.15b).

5. Explosively extend the arms to throw the ball straight up for the partner to catch. The goal is a short amortization phase (pause between the eccentric and concentric phases) after an enhanced eccentric phase (ball being dropped and moved to chest) (figure 5.15c).

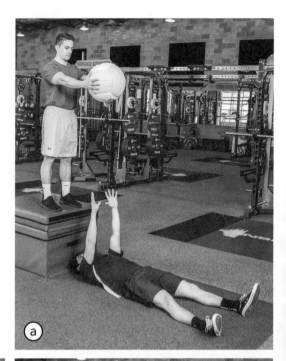
(a)

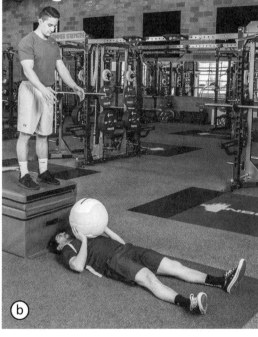
(b)

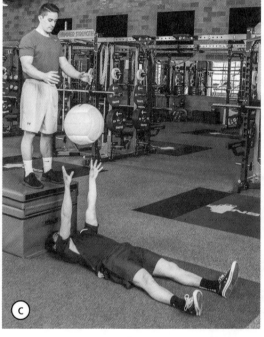
(c)

Figure 5.15 Ball drop throw at (a) the start position, (b) at the end of the countermovement, and (c) after the ballistic concentric action.

ABDOMINAL TWIST

Level: Advanced

Action

1. Begin by siting on the ground with the hips and knees flexed and the feet flat on the ground.
2. The starting position is the end of the concentric portion of an abdominal crunch with a twist to the right.
3. In the starting position, hold onto a standard medicine ball or bumper plate with the arms nearly fully extended (figure 5.16a).
4. Rapidly twist to the left, keeping the arms nearly fully extended so that the ball travels in an arc over the body and makes contact with the ground on the left side (figure 5.16b).
5. Repeat this movement back to the right side for one complete repetition.

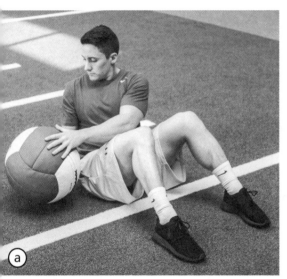 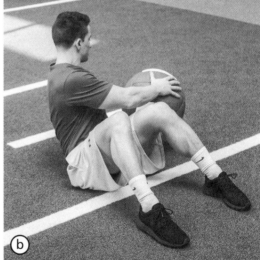

Figure 5.16 Abdominal twist at (a) the start position and (b) during the concentric action.

Variations

This exercise can also be performed with a rope power ball. In that variation, allow the ball to take a small bounce to create a short amortization phase to decrease the need to decelerate the ball toward the end of the movement (which is what an athlete needs to do when holding a standard medicine ball or bumper plate).

CONCLUSION

Developing upper body power is complex. Coaches and athletes should consider the athlete's level (novice, intermediate, advanced) when programming and choosing exercises. In addition, several training aids may enhance the intrinsic properties of power development, such as elastic bands and plyometric exercise. However, the literature neither presents a clear picture of the long-term effects of using these aids nor offers concrete evidence on establishing training intensity. Currently, applied recommendations include training at 30%-60% of 1RM for optimal power development and using both ballistic and plyometric exercises in training. In addition, establishing a strength base in both the upper and lower body may lead to reduction of injury and greater improvement in transfer of momentum for sport-specific activities like ball passing, pitching, and stick shooting.

CHAPTER 6

Lower Body Power Exercises

Jeremy M. Sheppard,
PhD, CSCS

Lower body power is a critical athletic quality for many sports. Depending on the sport, lower body power may be expressed through a variety of activities. Vertical jumping with and without a run-up (e.g., volleyball, basketball, high jump) is a common expression and assessment of lower body power. However, well-developed lower body power is required for acceleration and speed in every running sport, as well as for sports that require locomotion through the lower body (e.g., ice hockey, cycling, skiing, board sports). Coaches and athletes should consider the unique demands of these tasks in training. High-force, lower body power is also important for tackles (e.g., rugby, football) and any other task requiring locomotion against a heavy resistance (e.g., bobsled start, rugby scrum). Athletes can choose from a spectrum of exercises depending on the athletes' needs and the sporting application.

Effective lower body power should not be seen solely as a means to quickly *apply* force; one must develop power and skill to also effectively *absorb* force. With this application in mind, specific training should also be aimed at developing power and skill in the landing task and learning to reduce force in a graduated manner. In a landing, this is ideally conducted with the knees aligned over feet, not inward, and with the torso within the base of support, not collapsed with the chest over the toes.

To be effective in other sporting contexts, the force absorption is part of a rapid stretch-shortening cycle (SSC) (e.g., running and changing direction in football) and subsequent concentric movement. For these contexts, rapid SSC plyometric activities that train the cycle of force absorption and force production are warranted for performance. However, it is critical for all sports to develop fundamental lower body power for absorbing force, regardless of whether the time to absorb the force is relatively long (e.g., gymnasts landing from a high bar) or short (e.g., rapid cutting maneuver in football). It should be a fundamental movement quality in training programs. In addition, proper alignment of the body segments to reduce injury and optimize performance is critical and must be implemented for all exercises.

This chapter outlines key exercises that lead to superior lower body power performance. To optimize the application of the information, however, view and interpret this chapter in concert with others, particularly chapters 5 and 7 (including Olympic weightlifting and whole-body medicine ball work) because these training methods are highly effective for lower body power development as well as for force absorption. For ease of reference, the exercises in this chapter are organized into three categories based on their primary purpose: force-absorption exercises, plyometric exercises, and ballistic exercises.

FORCE-ABSORPTION EXERCISES

Learning to absorb force through landing and stabilizing is part of an effective training program. In fact, for jumping sports, it is most sensible to prioritize landing technique *before* emphasizing other aspects of jump training. For sports that rely on rapid changes of direction, developing proper mechanics and power in absorbing force is critical to injury prevention and performance. Prioritizing skills in this order ensures that athletes are technically and more physically prepared to tolerate the high demands of landing and cutting motions. In all contexts, athletes should aim to develop effective biomotor abilities, placing particular emphasis on control, motion, and strength from the earliest age possible (see chapter 4), to ensure that proper structural strength, stability, range, and movement are developed for the relevant force-absorption task.

Much of the benefit of force-absorption exercises is related to the ability to control body position and absorb force. These skills require regular attention, lending themselves to nearly daily practice of a few quality sets of low repetitions (1-2 exercises, 2-3 sets, 2-3 repetitions). The total volume is not large because although these are considered skill exercises, the force generated in some exercises, particularly altitude landings, can be relatively high. With this in mind, movement quality is the paramount consideration when increasing drop heights, volumes, and complexity.

ALTITUDE LANDING

Purpose

An altitude landing is a drop and stick to develop bilateral landing ability.

Action

1. Drop from a box by stepping out and absorbing the landing force primarily through an active ankle, knee, and hip action. The torso is centered within the base of support (figure 6.1).

2. The landing should be relatively quiet, as a reflection of peak force absorption.

3. Drop heights should only be increased by small (e.g. 10 cm or 4 in) magnitudes, from 20 cm (8 in), to 30 cm (12 in), based on movement competency, with likely upper limits of 70 to 80 cm (28-31 in) appropriate for most athletes.

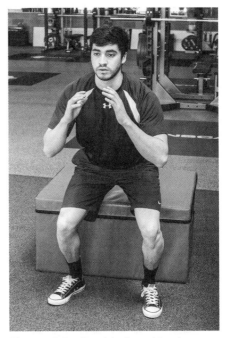

Figure 6.1 Double-leg altitude landing.

SINGLE-LEG ALTITUDE LANDING

Purpose

To develop the ability to land on one leg.

Action

1. Perform this the same as the altitude landing, but land on one leg instead of both (figure 6.2).

2. Use conservative drop heights, beginning with 10 cm (4 in) and progressions of 5-10 cm (2-4 in) up to ~40 cm (16 in) only when the athlete demonstrates excellent landing competency.

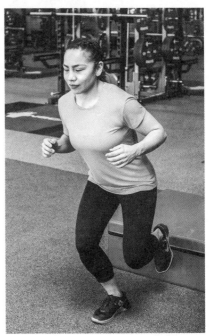

Figure 6.2 Single-leg altitude landing.

FORWARD HOP AND STICK

Purpose

To develop the ability to absorb force in a landing from a horizontal plane.

Action

1. Perform a double-leg forward hop (figure 6.3a), absorbing the force with a double-leg stick (figure 6.3b).

2. The athlete can also perform a double-leg forward hop with a single-leg landing (figure 6.3c).

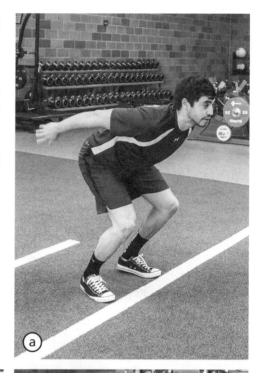

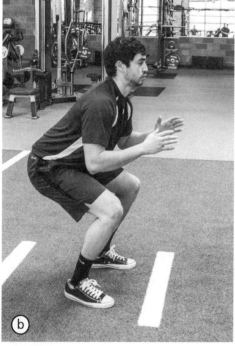

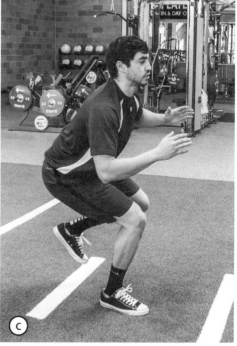

Figure 6.3 Forward hop starting position (a) and stick landing on two legs (b) and on one leg (c).

TRIPLE AND PENTA HOP AND STICK

Purpose

This exercise expands on the forward hop and stick by increasing the demand to develop the ability to absorb force in a landing from a horizontal plane with higher velocity.

Action

1. In the triple, perform two ballistic hops and then stick the final landing. In the penta hop, perform four ballistic hops and then stick the fifth contact.

2. Variations include a double-leg hop and stick with a double-leg landing (figure 6.4a) and a double-leg forward hop with a single-leg landing (figure 6.4b).

3. The athlete can also perform single-leg hops throughout (figure 6.4c).

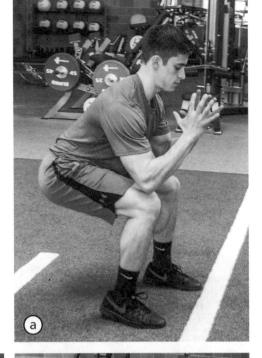

Figure 6.4 (a) Double-leg hop and stick with a double-leg landing, (b) double-leg forward hop with single-leg landing, and (c) single-leg hop variation.

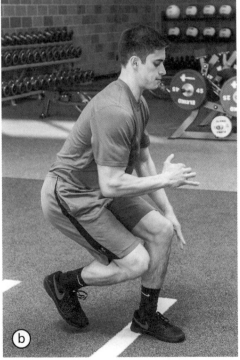

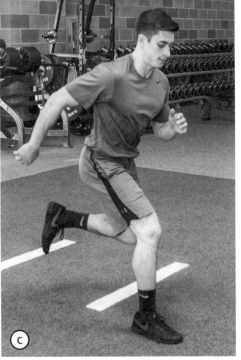

LATERAL HOP AND STICK

Purpose
To develop the ability to absorb force in a landing from a lateral movement.

Action
1. Perform a simple double-leg lateral hop (figure 6.5a) and absorb the force with a double-leg stick (figure 6.5b).
2. Alternatively, performed as a double-leg lateral hop with a single-leg landing.

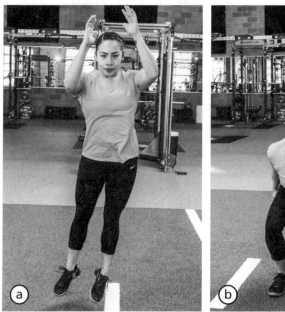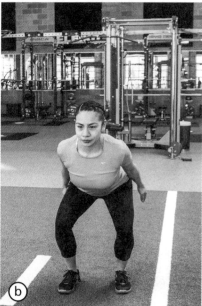

Figure 6.5 Lateral hop and stick. (a) Double-leg lateral hop and (b) double-leg stick.

ZIG-ZAG WITH STICK

Purpose
The athlete performs lateral bounds in a zig-zag pattern, sticking each landing to develop control and coordination.

Action
1. Hold each landing for 2-3 s before bounding into the next movement (figure 6.6). This emphasizes control.
2. To make the exercise more fluid, pause only briefly in each position.

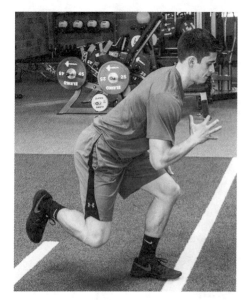

Figure 6.6 Zig-zag with stick.

TRIPLE AND PENTA LATERAL HOP AND STICK

Purpose

This exercise expands on the lateral hop and stick by increasing the demand to develop the ability to absorb force in a landing in the lateral direction with higher velocity.

Action

1. In the triple, perform two lateral ballistic hops and then stick the final landing. In the penta hop, perform four lateral ballistic hops and stick the fifth contact.
2. Variations include a double-leg hop and stick with a double-leg landing (figure 6.7a) and a double-leg lateral hop with a single-leg landing (figure 6.7b).
3. The athlete can also perform single-leg lateral hops throughout (figure 6.7c).

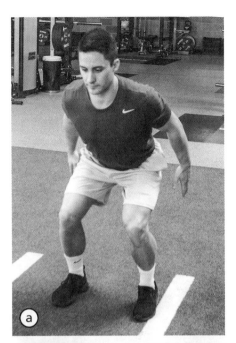
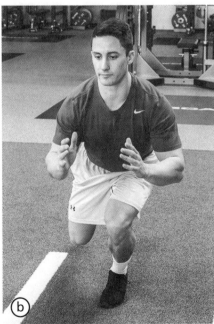
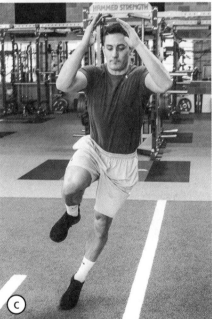

Figure 6.7 Triple and penta lateral hop and stick with (a) double-leg landing, (b) double-leg lateral hop with a single-leg landing, and (c) single-leg lateral hop variation.

LATERAL ALTITUDE LANDING

Purpose

Lateral altitude landings are a sideways drop and stick on a single leg to develop lateral landing ability.

Action

1. Drop from a low box by stepping out and absorbing the landing force primarily through an active ankle, knee, and hip action (figure 6.8a-b). The torso is centered within the base of support.
2. The landing should be relatively quiet as a reflection of peak force absorption.
3. Start with a drop height of 10 cm (4 in) and increase cautiously in modest increments to 30-40 cm (12-16 in) based on the athlete's movement competency.

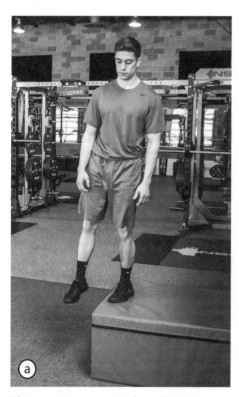 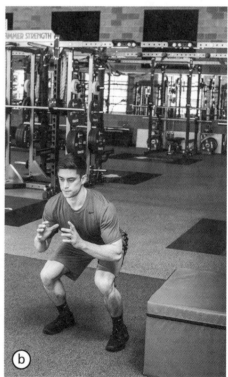

Figure 6.8 Lateral altitude landing.

PLYOMETRIC EXERCISES

Plyometric training emphasizes a rapid transition from eccentric (net muscle lengthening) to concentric (net muscle shortening) movement (termed the *SSC*). Include this type of training in a program to develop lower body power, particularly for sports that require this rapid transition (e.g., jumping, cutting, running).

In SSC-based movements, the eccentric force, reflex stimuli, and elastic contribution are greater than normal because of the eccentric (stretch) load. In training settings, this can be magnified even further with accentuated eccentric SSC activities such as depth jumps. For example, high-velocity tuck jumps are an overloaded eccentric movement because the athlete rapidly extends the legs downward from a tuck position to jump explosively again. Hence, the rate at which the feet contact the ground is greater than normal, or accentuated.

Plyometric exercises should develop an attribute required for sport, such as power or strength, and should not necessarily mimic a sport movement. However, plyometric exercises should be used to develop the SSC ability that is *relevant* to a sport-specific movement. For example, elite volleyball players may perform countermovement-style jumps (block jumps, jump sets, and spike jumps) 1,000 to 4,000 times per week simply through practice and matches. Adding a few sets of countermovement jumps (CMJs) will only add to an already large load of the same jump. The strength and conditioning coach must therefore carefully consider the use and purpose of plyometric training and target a specific physical quality (e.g., accentuated eccentrics, ballistic exercises, maximal strength training, recovery and regeneration) based on the athlete's needs and other training considerations.

Plyometric exercises are extremely effective. However, this does not mean that more is better. On the contrary, low frequency (2-3 sessions per week) and low volume (3-6 sets of 2-5 repetitions) are most appropriate. It is not necessary to perform myriad plyometric exercises. Getting the most out of a program requires mastering the movements of the exercises themselves. For most athletes, two or three plyometric exercises at any one time is sufficient for attaining movement mastery and obtaining considerable benefit.

JUMP SQUAT

Purpose

To develop lower body power using the stretch-shortening cycle.

Action

1. The jump squat, or vertical jump, is typically performed with a countermovement, and is commonly known as the CMJ.
2. Begin in a standing position with the feet approximately shoulder-width apart.
3. Initiate the countermovement by dropping to a self-selected position (figure 6.9a). Then, immediately jump off the ground (figure 6.9b).
4. Perform the jump with or without an arm swing.

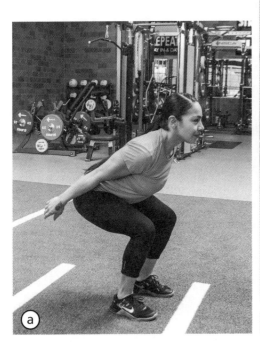
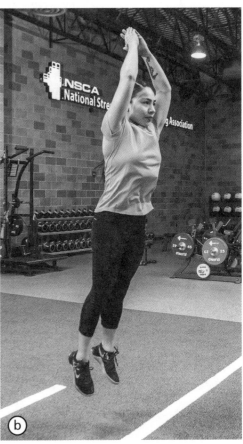

Figure 6.9 Jump squat (a) squatting to the self-selected position and (b) jumping.

SQUAT JUMP

Purpose
To develop lower body power.

Action

1. Pause during the squat jump at a set angle to ensure that this is not an SSC activity and instead relies on pure concentric power.

2. One variation is to hold the bottom position for 2-3 s (figure 6.10a).

3. The athlete can also pause on a box before jumping as high as possible (figure 6.10b).

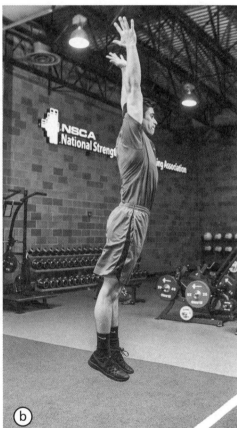

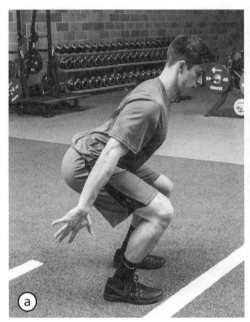

Figure 6.10 Squat jump (a) holding the bottom position and (b) jumping as high as possible.

TUCK JUMP

Purpose
To develop lower body power.

Action

1. To initiate the tuck jump, perform a vertical jump as high as possible, and then tuck the knees up so that the thighs are vertical (figure 6.11a-b).

2. As the athlete descends, extend the legs downward, increasing the speed of the impact from the initial jump.

3. Repeat jumping, tucking, and extending the legs, creating a greater than normal impact and fast, explosive contact with the ground.

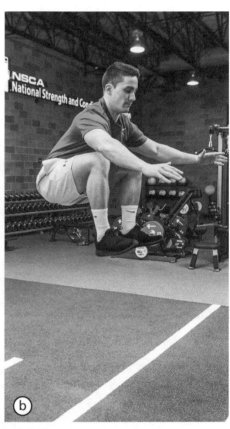

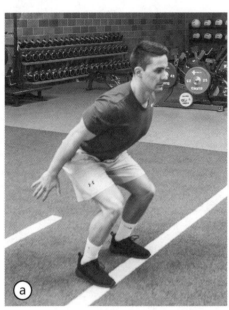

Figure 6.11 Tuck jump (a) start position and (b) jump.

SINGLE-LEG TUCK JUMP

Purpose
To develop lower body power.

Action

1. This is performed similarly to a tuck jump but requires considerably more strength and skill to be performed on a single leg.

2. Initiate the first double-leg jump.

3. Immediately land and jump using a single-leg landing and takeoff.

DEPTH JUMP

Purpose

Depth jumps are a specific method of accentuated eccentric overload to develop lower body power. The height of the drop provides a greater than normal eccentric load. The ability to use this extra eccentric load to improve concentric performance (i.e., impulse and jump height) is a diagnostic tool sometimes called *stretch load tolerance*.

Action

1. Begin by standing on a box or platform.
2. Step off the box and drop to the ground and jump as high as possible. This emphasizes the highest impulse (figure 6.12a-b).
3. The optimal drop height is one that elicits the greatest jump height. Athletes can experiment with a range of heights (e.g. 10-50 cm or 4 to 20 in) to determine the height that elicits their highest jump performance. Perform the exercise from that optimal height, and also from 10 cm (4 in) higher than optimal.

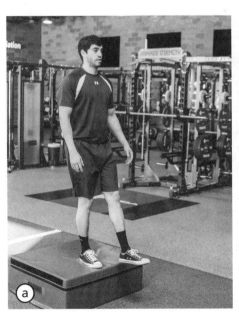
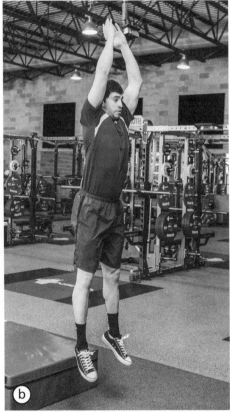

Figure 6.12 Depth jump *(a)* stepping off box and *(b)* jumping as high as possible.

Variation

In a bounce depth jump, drop from a lower height (typically 25%-50% lower than the depth jump) and attempt to use a minimal ground contact time.

ACCENTUATED ECCENTRIC LOADED JUMP

Purpose
This exercise uses a handheld load to provide additional stimulation through the eccentric action of a jump.

Action

1. Stand with feet shoulder-width apart and arms extended at the sides, while holding a dumbbell in each hand (for a total additional load of 20-40% of body-mass). Flex the knees and lower the dumbbells toward the ground (figure 6.13a).

2. Drop the dumbbells at the bottom body position during the transition from the eccentric action to the concentric movement of the jump and then jump explosively (figure 6.13b). Ideally, this is a rhythmic movement.

3. The additional lengthening load provides a greater than normal myogenic (muscular) setup for the subsequent concentric (shortening) load in the jump.

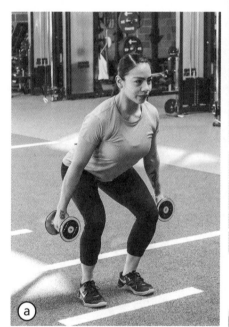
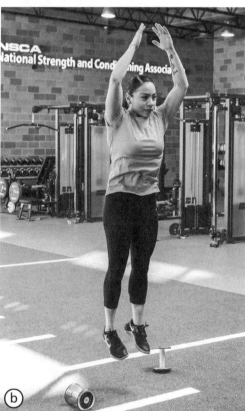

Figure 6.13 Accentuated eccentric loaded jump (a) just before dropping the load and (b) jumping as high as possible.

ASSISTED JUMP

Purpose

To provide an overspeed stimulus and long-term adaptions to jump velocity.

Action

1. Begin in a standing position using handheld powerlifting bands or bungee cords in a harness (figure 6.14a).

2. Descend by squatting down into the countermovement of the jump, while stretching the bands or bungee cords, which provide assistance during the concentric phase of the jump (figure 6.14b).

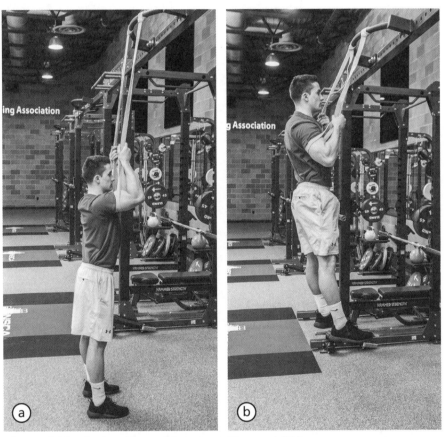

Figure 6.14 Assisted jump (a) start position and (b) jump.

BOX JUMP

Purpose

This exercise reduces the peak landing force because the athlete jumps up to land.

Action

1. Stand facing a box (figure 6.15a). The height of the box will depend on the athlete's capabilities.
2. Jump from the ground onto the box from both feet and land on both feet (figure 6.15b).

Note: A criticism of this exercise is that it does not follow a movement pattern found in very many sports; however, some sports, such as surfing, skateboarding, snow boarding, parkour, and Olympic lifting, include jumps and lower body extension followed by a tuck. Athletes and coaches should consider their specific requirements and the potential benefits of reducing landing load in the context of their sport.

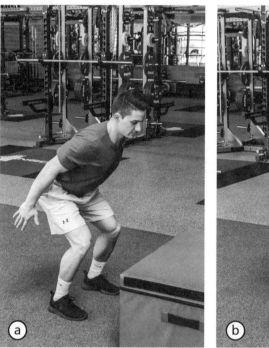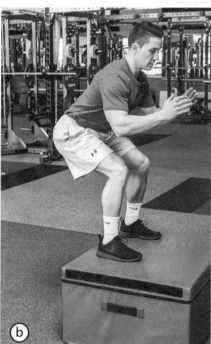

Figure 6.15 Box jump (a) squat position and (b) landing.

DEPTH JUMP TO BOX JUMP

Purpose

To gain the benefits of a depth jump while reducing the subsequent landing force.

Action

1. Start by standing on the edge of the first box, and prepare to drop by stepping forward with the front foot off the box and the back foot still on the box (figure 6.16a).

2. Drop from the prescribed height (figure 6.16b).

3. Immediately jump maximally to land on the second box (figure 6.16c). The height of both the box and the drop will depend on the athlete's capabilities.

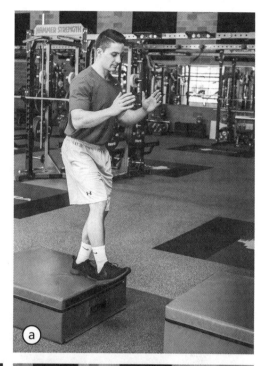

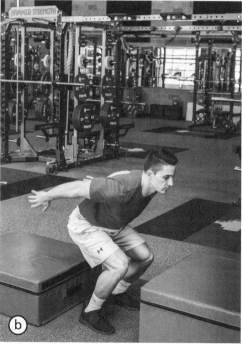

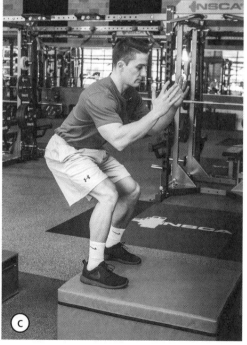

Figure 6.16 Depth jump to box jump (a) start position, (b) initial landing, and (c) box landing.

SPLIT JUMP

Purpose
To develop lower body power from a lunge position.

Action

1. Begin by standing in a split stance (lunge) (figure 6.17a).
2. Jump upward and switch the stance (opposite leg is forward) repeatedly for the prescribed number of repetitions (figure 6.17b).

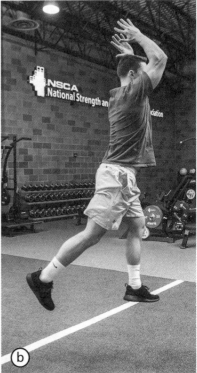
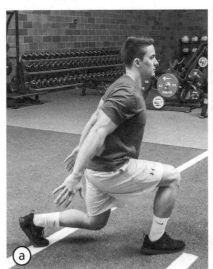

Figure 6.17 Split jump (a) lunge position and (b) jump.

ANKLE BOUNCE (POGO)

Purpose
To develop lower body power and stiffness.

Action

1. Standing upright, jump upward, propelling the body primarily from ankle stiffness while actively dorsiflexing the ankle.
2. Use minimal knee and hip bend to pogo up and down (figure 6.18).

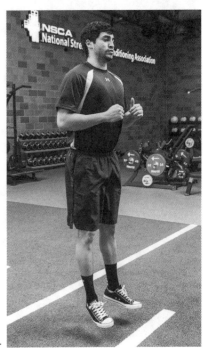

Figure 6.18 Ankle bounces (pogos).

BROAD JUMP

Purpose

To develop lower body horizontal power.

Action

1. The broad jump, or horizontal jump, is typically performed with a countermovement initiated from an upright stance with the feet parallel and with an active arm swing.
2. Jump forward as far as possible and land on both feet (figure 6.19).

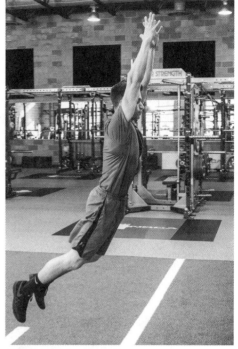

Figure 6.19 Broad jump.

HALTERE-LOADED REPEATED BROAD JUMP

Purpose

The increased jump distance and use of handheld weights provide an additional load during the eccentric phase. Broad jumps performed with halteres (handheld weights of ancient Greece) are one of the oldest known training methods.

Action

1. Perform this exercise similarly to the previous broad jump while holding a dumbbell in each hand (figure 6.20). Begin with low loads of just a few kilograms per dumbbell.
2. The handheld weight provides additional momentum through the arm swing. Therefore, the athlete will travel a greater distance than in the standard broad jump, and the athlete must absorb more force in the landing of each jump before proceeding into the next.
3. Repeat the movement by immediately springing forward after landing on both feet for the required number of repetitions.

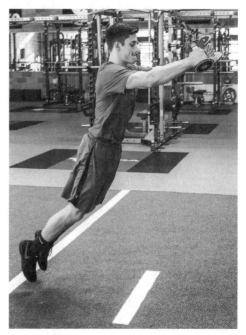

Figure 6.20 Haltere-loaded repeated broad jump.

DEPTH JUMP TO BROAD JUMP

Purpose
To develop vertical and horizontal power in the lower body.

Action

1. Begin by performing a depth jump.
2. Immediately after landing, perform a double-leg broad jump.

Variations
Variations can include horizontal single-leg hops (from markedly lower heights) from a depth jump or a depth jump into a sprint acceleration.

DOUBLE-LEG HOP

Purpose
To develop lower body horizontal power.

Action

1. Begin by performing a depth jump (figure 6.21a-b).
2. Repeat this sequence for the prescribed repetitions.

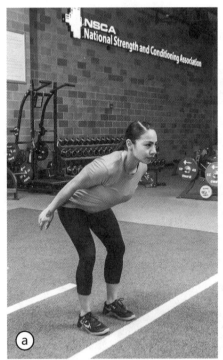
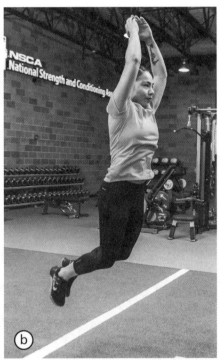

Figure 6.21 Double-leg hop (a) start position and (b) jump.

Variations
Perform the repeated hop on one leg. The athlete can perform both single- and double-leg hops for a specific number of repetitions and then break into a sprint acceleration (e.g., 5 hops followed by a 20 m [22 yd] sprint acceleration).

INCLINE HOP

Purpose

Performing the double-leg hop on an incline increases the amount of propulsive drive and lower body horizontal power developed.

Action

1. Stand at the bottom of an incline and prepare to perform double-leg hops up the incline.
2. Hop for the prescribed number of repetitions.

BOUNDING

Purpose

To develop lower body horizontal power.

Action

1. Bounding is a striding exercise performed on alternating legs (figure 6.22a-b).
2. Work to optimize flight time during this exercise.
3. The typical distance for this exercise is 20-40 m (22-44 yd), but can be extended to develop greater endurance.

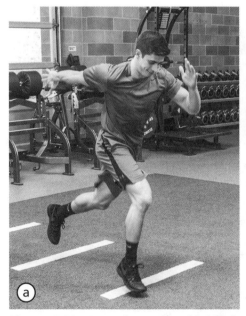 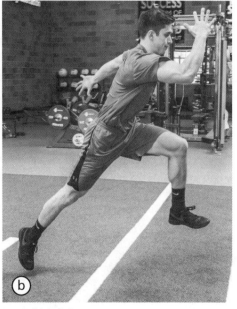

Figure 6.22 Bounding on the (a) right leg and (b) left leg.

INCLINE BOUNDING

Purpose

To develop lower body horizontal power while reducing landing impact. The incline provides further resistance and reduces the impact of the landing.

Action

1. Perform the standard bounding exercise on a slight incline.
2. The typical distance for this exercise is 20-30 m (22-33 yd) but can be extended to develop greater endurance.

ZIG-ZAG BOUNDING

Purpose

To develop lower body horizontal and lateral power by incorporating a lateral zig-zag pattern. This exercise has also been termed a skater's bound as it resembles the movement pattern of ice skating.

Action

1. Bound both forward and laterally from foot to foot as quickly and explosively as possible (figure 6.23a-b).
2. The typical distance for this exercise is 20-40 m (22-44 yd).

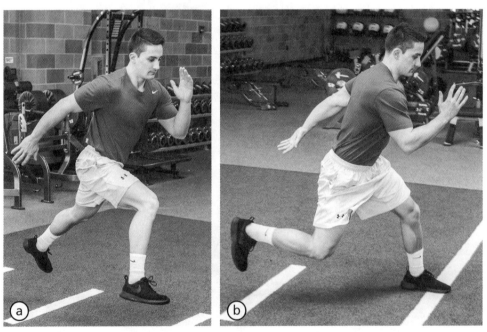

Figure 6.23 Zig-zag bounding on the (a) right leg and (b) left leg.

BALLISTIC EXERCISES

Ballistic exercise refers to the category of movements that applies resistance beyond body weight. These exercises are at an intermediate to an advanced level and should be performed only after the athlete is able to perform exercises such as the jump squat or CMJ correctly. The loads are generally light enough to allow movement more rapid than that of near-maximal heavy-resistance training and Olympic weightlifting (although these methods are important for power development). Ballistic exercises offer a range of loads from which to target the force–velocity spectrum. While heavy-resistance training targets maximal force capability, and plyometric training targets fast SSC activity against a relatively low load, ballistic exercise develops power against moderate loads. Ballistic exercise offers the athlete a high rate of force development.

Jump variations with load are the most common lower body ballistic exercise. These can be conducted with SSC involvement (CMJ) or without SSC contribution to attend to specific sport demands. Accentuated eccentric loaded jump squats (extra load in the descend phase) are also an effective and relatively common exercise for developing lower body power because the additional stimuli in the eccentric action yields a greater than normal concentric power output.

Squat movements (e.g., back squat, front squat) are considered maximal strength exercises. However, reducing the bar load by 20%-50% while applying an accommodating resistance through the use of powerlifting bands or heavy chains increases the acceleration phase, compared to normal conditions. Whether the band stretches or the chain unfurls off of the floor during the concentric action, the resistance increases throughout the concentric part of the movement. Therefore, the athlete has to exert force through a much longer period. As a result, this this movement becomes a highly effective lower body power exercise.

Practitioners can program ballistic exercises within a training week in several ways. One method is to dedicate a single training session per week for all ballistic exercises, performing 5-6 exercises, 3-5 sets each, with 3-5 repetitions. Another method is to complete lower volumes of ballistic exercise (1-2 exercises, 3-5 repetitions) more frequently within the week or at each training session (2-5 sessions per week). Specific programming examples are given in chapters 9 and 10. Regardless, as with all velocity-based training, attention to quality of movement and output (power and velocity under load) is paramount to success.

BACK SQUAT

Purpose
To develop lower body strength and power.

Action

1. Begin by gripping the bar with a shoulder-width pronated grip and placing it on the upper back and shoulders (high-bar or low-bar position can be used). The toes point slightly outward, the chest is out, and the head is tilted slightly upward (figure 6.24a).

2. Descend by flexing the hips and knees while maintaining a neutral back position until the desired position is reached. This is usually when the thighs are parallel to the floor (figure 6.24b).

3. Return to the starting position by extending the hips and knees while maintaining a neutral back position.

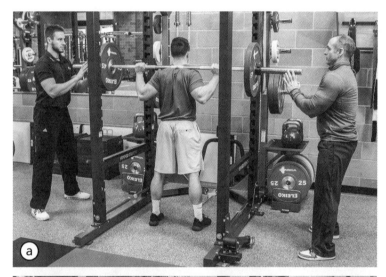

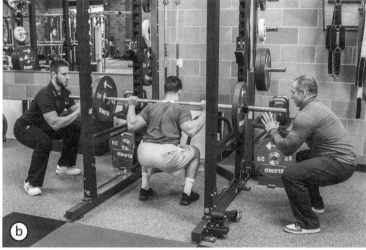

Figure 6.24 Back squat (a) start position and (b) bottom position.

FRONT SQUAT

Purpose

To develop lower body strength and power.

Action

1. Begin with the bar placed across the front of the shoulders (using either the parallel-arm or crossed-arm position). The chest is up and out and the head is tilted slightly upward (figure 6.25a).
2. Descend by flexing the hips and the knees while maintaining a neutral back position until the desired position is reached. This is usually when the thighs are parallel to the floor (figure 6.25b).
3. Return to the starting position by extending the hips and knees while maintaining a neutral back position.

Note: When performing the back and front squat, consider safety and proper technique. Use two spotters, one at each end of the bar.

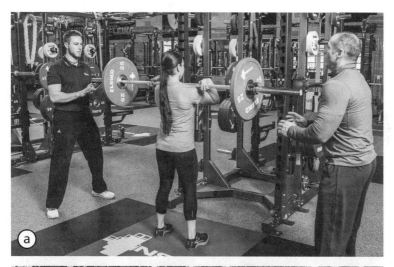

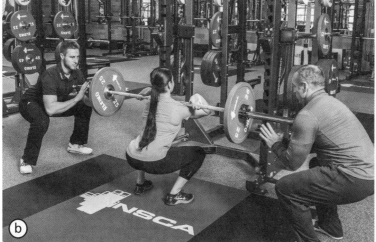

Figure 6.25   Front squat *(a)* start position and *(b)* bottom position.

LOADED JUMP SQUAT

Purpose

To develop lower body power using the SSC and to develop the ability to tolerate an external load.

Action

1. Loaded jump squats are a fluid countermovement jumps performed with a load from a barbell or a weighted vest. The load is typically 10%-50% of body mass. In some cases the load is much greater to try to match the higher force demands of powerful movement in that sport (e.g., track sprint cycling, football linemen).
2. Descend and then transition to a vertical jump (figure 6.26a-b).

Note: When performing loaded jumps with a barbell, proper technique is critical for safety, so make sure that excellent form is well established in unloaded jump squats before progressing to using loads.

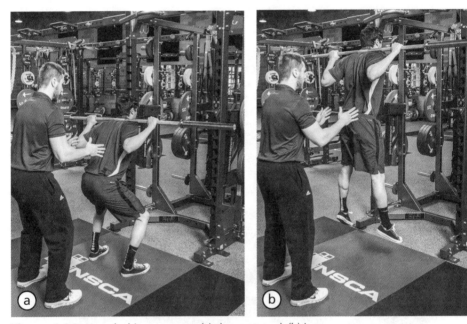

Figure 6.26 Loaded jump squat (a) descent and (b) jump.

LOADED SQUAT JUMP

Purpose

This exercise develops lower body power and the ability to tolerate external loads without using the SSC.

Action

1. The load, which is usually 10%-50% of body mass, can be applied using a barbell or a weighted vest. In some cases, much greater loads are used.
2. Descend and pause at the bottom position for 2-3 seconds, before transitioning to a vertical jump.

Note: When performing loaded jumps with a barbell, keep safety and proper technique in mind. Use a spotter for these exercises.

BAND OR CHAIN SQUAT

Purpose

To develop lower body strength and power.

Action

1. Perform a front or back squat using a barbell load reduced by 20%-50% of the load the athlete usually uses for a specific rep scheme. Additional accommodating resistance is added through the use of heavy-duty bands or chains.
2. The additional load will prolong the length of time that the athlete accelerates the load.
3. The load selected for the barbell and for the band (the thickness) or chains (the weight) should reflect the emphasis desired. Lighter loads allow greater movement speed, and heavier loads develop greater force.

Note: This method is described in more detail in chapter 8.

ACCENTUATED ECCENTRIC LOADED BOX JUMP SQUAT

Purpose

To develop lower body power using the SSC and the ability to tolerate an eccentric load.

Action

1. Use dumbbells (15%-25% of body weight) to overload the eccentric (drop) phase in a jump.

2. Drop the dumbbells at the bottom position during the shift from an eccentric to a concentric action, and then jump on to the top of the box (figure 6.27a-c).

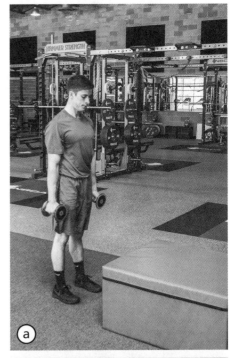

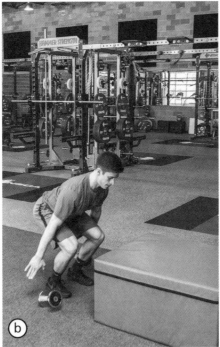

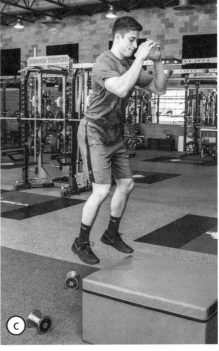

Figure 6.27 Accentuated eccentric loaded box jump squat *(a)* start position, *(b)* release of dumbbells, and *(c)* jump onto box.

SLED PULL

Purpose

To develop lower body horizontal power.

Action

1. Sled pulls require a harness and a loadable sled the athlete will pull while accelerating into a sprint (figure 6.28).
2. Choose the load and distance depending on the athlete's goal. Shorter distances (e.g. 10-30 m [11-33 yd]) allow a high-quality effort. The load should not be so heavy that running mechanics deteriorate.

Note: The friction between the sled and the ground will affect the load.

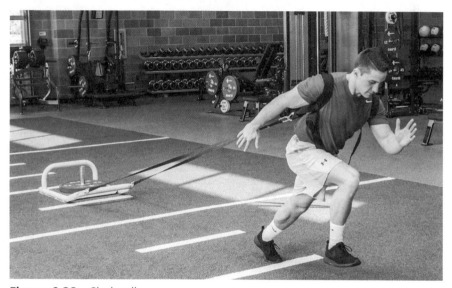

Figure 6.28   Sled pull.

SLED PUSH

Purpose
To develop lower body horizontal power.

Action

1. This exercise is similar to the sled pull, but the athlete accelerates the sled by pushing it (figure 6.29).
2. This variation is suitable for sports in which horizontal leg power is applied without driving the arms (American football, rugby).

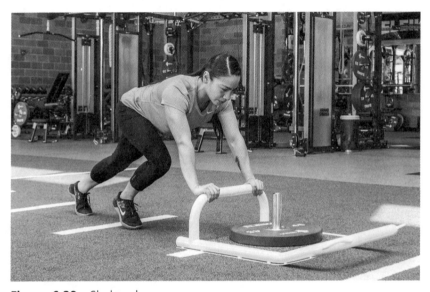

Figure 6.29   Sled push.

RESISTED LATERAL AND MULTIDIRECTIONAL ACCELERATION

Purpose

To develop multidirectional lower body power.

Action

1. Using a powerlifting band around the waist and held by a partner, or a harness attached to resistance, perform movements such as lateral shuffles for basketball or lateral lunge steps for volleyball. Maintain a sport-relevant posture (figure 6.30).
2. Perform backward movements such as those for a football defensive back and movements that combine forward, lateral, and backward movement such as those found in soccer, rugby, and American football.

Note: The distance covered depends on the sport.

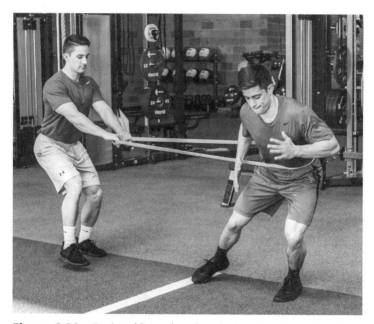

Figure 6.30   Resisted lateral and multidirectional acceleration.

CONCLUSION

There are a myriad of effective power development methods for the lower body. When selecting exercises and approaches, it is important to consider two main factors. First, one must consider the sporting context, so that training efforts are relevant to the task in the sport. Second, it is important to consider the main areas of improvement potential for the individual athlete by understanding their strengths and weaknesses. Considering these two factors in concert with each other will drive making decisions and designing programs for lower body power development.

Total Body Power Exercises

Adam Storey, PhD

The sport of competitive weightlifting requires two multijoint, total body exercises to be performed in competition: the snatch and the clean and jerk. These exercises require athletes to exert high forces in an explosive manner in order to lift the barbell from the floor to an overhead position or to the shoulders in one continuous movement. During the performance of these exercises, weightlifters have achieved some of the highest absolute and relative peak power outputs reported in the literature (8-11).

Although the two competitive exercises form the basis of the training programs for competitive weightlifters, several complementary exercises that have movement patterns similar to the competitive exercises (e.g., power snatch and power snatch from hang, power clean and power clean from hang, snatch and clean pull, front and back squat) are also included in training (16). These complementary exercises are routinely incorporated into the training programs of other strength and power athletes because of the kinematic similarities that exist between the propulsive phases in both weightlifting and jumping movements (i.e., the explosive ankle, knee, and hip extension) (2, 3, 6, 7, 12, 13). They are also frequently used because of the significant relationships that exist between weightlifting ability in these exercises and power output during jumping and sprinting (1, 3, 4, 13, 17) and tests of agility (13).

During the snatch and the clean and jerk, weightlifters have been shown to produce peak power at loads of 70%-80% of 1RM (5, 14, 15), which demonstrates an improved ability to generate peak power under high-load conditions. As such, other athletes who are required to generate high peak power outputs against heavy external loads (e.g., wrestlers, bobsledders, and rugby and American football players) are likely to benefit from high-load, weightlifting-style training.

This chapter details the purpose and teaching progressions for total body power exercises that are derived from weightlifting. Because of the high-speed nature and complexity of these movements, inexperienced lifters should seek the guidance of a certified strength and conditioning specialist when attempting to learn these lifting progressions. In addition, lifters should make sure they can perform these exercises correctly before increasing the load.

KEY ASPECTS FOR THE TOTAL BODY POWER EXERCISE PROGRESSIONS

The exercises outlined in this chapter are described using the following terms and positions.

Hook Grip

When gripping the barbell, the index and middle fingers wrap over the top of the thumb in order to apply pressure to both the thumb and the barbell (figure 7.1). The hook grip minimizes the chance that an athlete's grip will fail during the explosive pulling phase of the Olympic lifts.

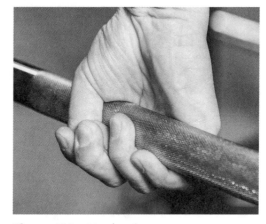

Figure 7.1 Hook grip.

Grip Placement for the Snatch-Related Exercises

During the snatch-related exercises, use a wide overhand (also known as pronated) or snatch grip. The width of the grip depends on several factors, including the athlete's arm length, shoulder flexibility, and injury status. A simple method to determine the optimal width for the snatch grip is to measure the length from the outside of the shoulder to the end of a closed fist on the opposite arm, which is abducted from the body at 90° (figure 7.2). The measured distanced corresponds to the distance between the index fingers when gripping the barbell for the snatch-related exercises. An alternative is the elbow-to-elbow method (also known as the scarecrow method).

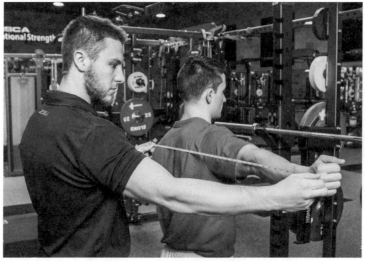

Figure 7.2 Measuring the optimal width for the snatch grip.

Straight-Arm Overhead Receiving Position

In the straight-arm overhead receiving position, the barbell is positioned over and behind the athlete's ears. When viewed from the side, the athlete's ears should not be blocked from view by the arms (figure 7.3). The bar should be in the palm of the hands and the wrists slightly extended.

Power Variations

A power snatch and a power clean are classified as exercises that are caught in an above parallel thigh position. If the lifter descends below this parallel thigh position, the exercise is deemed to be a full squat snatch and a full squat clean, respectively. Although the full squat variations enable proficient athletes to lift approximately 20% more load, and is therefore the reason they are performed in Olympic weightlifting competitions, they require a greater degree of technical mastery, mobility and strength when compared to the power variations.

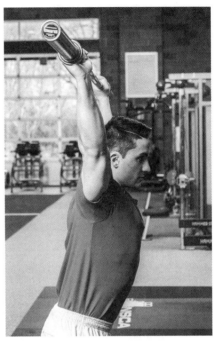

Figure 7.3   The overhead receiving position for the snatch and jerk-related progressions.

Hang Variations

The hang position refers to a starting position above knee. If an exercise is not described as using a hang position, assume that the movement is initiated from the floor.

Pull Variations

The pull variation of the snatch and clean exercises emphasizes the triple extension of the lower body, which is immediately followed by an explosive shoulder shrug. Except for the fast snatch and fast pull versions, the arms should remain relaxed and not actively engaged in an attempt to pull the bar upward; the elbows only flex after the athlete completes the lower body triple extension and upper body shrug. When the bar reaches its maximal height, it is not caught; instead, the athlete flexes the knees and hips and lowers the bar back to the starting position.

POWER SNATCH FROM HANG

Purpose

To develop explosive power in the vertical plane. This exercise is less technically demanding than the power snatch from floor.

Action

1. Using a wide overhand or a hook grip, begin by taking hold of a loaded barbell from a lifting rack (or set of blocks) set at midthigh height.
2. Position the feet between hip- and shoulder-width apart and facing forward.
3. Bend at the knees slightly and with a neutral spine, flex at the hips and lean the torso forward to allow the barbell to move down the thighs to a starting position just above the knees (i.e., hang position) (figure 7.4a). At this position, the shoulders should be over the barbell, the elbows pointed out to the sides, and the head facing forward.
4. Begin the movement by rapidly extending the hips, knees, and ankles while maintaining the shoulder position over the barbell.
5. Allow the barbell to slide up the thighs to ensure that it remains as close to the body as possible.
6. As the lower body joints reach full extension, rapidly shrug the shoulders.
7. When the shoulders reach their highest point, allow the elbows to flex to begin pulling the body under the barbell (figure 7.4b).
8. The explosive nature of this phase may cause the feet to lose contact with the floor.
9. Simultaneously flex the hips and knees into a quarter squat, and continue to pull the body below the barbell.
10. Once the body is under the bar, catch the bar in the straight-arm overhead receiving position described earlier.
11. Recover to a standing position while maintaining the barbell in the straight-arm overhead receiving position (figure 7.4c).
12. In a controlled fashion, lower the barbell by bending at the elbows and reducing the muscular tension in the shoulders. Simultaneously flex the hips and knees as the barbell is lowered to the thighs.

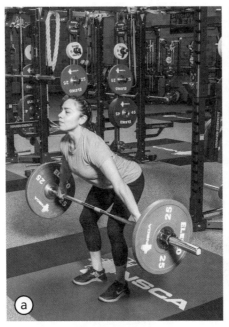

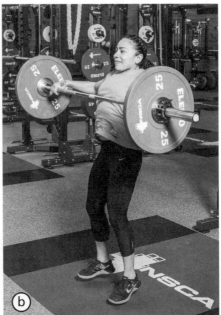

Figure 7.4 Power snatch from hang (a) start position, (b) movement with hip, knee, and ankle extension, and (c) recovery to a standing position.

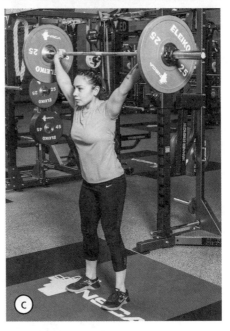

POWER SNATCH FROM BLOCKS

Purpose

To develop explosive power in the vertical plane using loads that are typically heavier than those used for the power snatch from hang. Conversely, one can use lighter loads from blocks to focus on the technical aspects of the exercise.

Action

1. Using a wide overhand or hook grip, begin with a loaded barbell on a set of lifting blocks. The height of the lifting blocks should position the barbell just above the knees.

2. At the starting position, the shoulders should be over the barbell, the elbows pointing out, and the head facing forward.

3. To complete the power snatch from blocks variation (figure 7.5a-c), refer to points 4-11 of the power snatch from hang.

4. In a controlled fashion, lower the barbell by bending at the elbows and reducing the muscular tension in the shoulders. Simultaneously flex the hips and knees as the barbell is lowered to the blocks.

Note: Use blocks of different heights to focus on different phases of the movement or to make the exercise more specific. For example, low blocks will allow a loaded barbell to be set from a starting position just below knee level, which will enable an individual to focus on the transition phase from the first pull (i.e. from the floor to below the knee) to the second pull (i.e. from above the knee to maximal hip and knee extension). Conversely, higher blocks will allow a loaded barbell to be set from a mid-thigh starting position which will enable an individual to emphasize a rapid hip and knee extension.

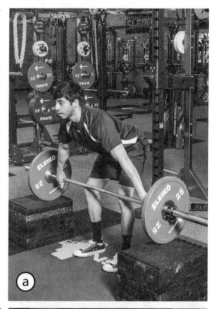
(a)

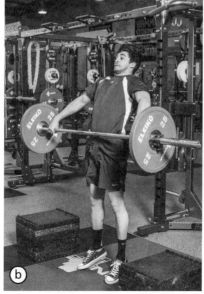
(b)

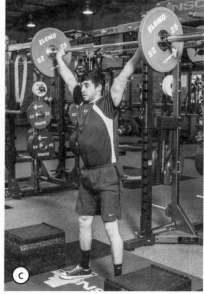
(c)

Figure 7.5 Power snatch from blocks.

POWER SNATCH FROM FLOOR

Purpose

To develop explosive power from the ground in the vertical plane.

Action

1. Begin with a loaded barbell on the ground.

2. From standing, position the barbell approximately a fist width from the shins and use a wide overhand or hook grip.

3. Position the heels between hip- and shoulder-width apart. The feet are slightly turned out.

4. To achieve an ideal starting position, lower the hips, elevate the chest, point the elbows out, direct the eyes slightly upward, and align the head with the spine. The shoulders must remain over the barbell in this set position while maintaining a neutral back (figure 7.6a).

5. Begin the movement by extending the hips and knees to lift the barbell off the floor while maintaining the barbell close to the shins. This initial phase of the exercise is termed the first pull. During this phase, maintain a neutral spine position, with the shoulders over the barbell. Do not let the hips rise before the shoulders rise; the torso-to-floor angle must be kept constant during this phase.

6. As the barbell rises above the knees, begin the second pull by moving the knees under the barbell so it slides up the thighs.

7. Rapidly extend the hips, knees, and ankles (triple extension) while the shoulders remain in line with the barbell and the elbows point out to the sides. The explosive nature of this phase may cause the feet to lose contact with the floor.

8. As the lower body joints reach full extension, rapidly shrug the shoulders (figure 7.6b).

9. When the shoulders reach their highest point, allow the elbows to flex to begin pulling the body under the barbell.

10. Simultaneously flex the hips and knees into a quarter-squat position while continuing to forcefully pull the body below the barbell.

11. Once the body is under the bar, catch the bar in the straight-arm overhead receiving position described earlier (figure 7.6c).

12. Recover to a standing position while maintaining the barbell in the straight-arm overhead receiving position (figure 7.6d).

13. In a controlled fashion, lower the barbell by bending at the elbows and reducing the muscular tension in the shoulders. Simultaneously flex the hips and knees as the barbell is lowered to the floor.

(continued)

POWER SNATCH FROM FLOOR *(continued)*

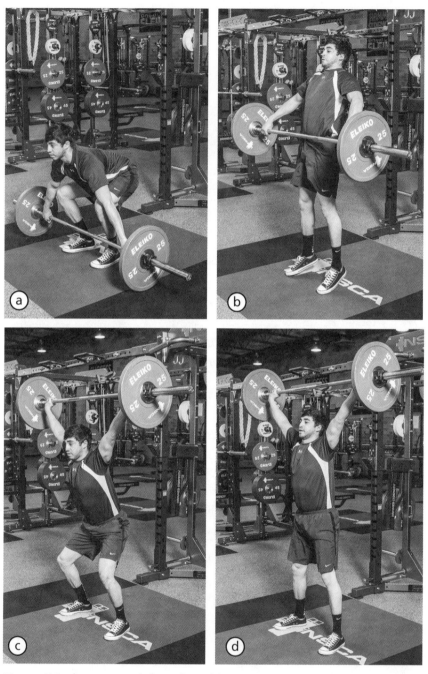

Figure 7.6 Power snatch from floor *(a)* start position, *(b)* triple extension, *(c)* catch, and *(d)* recovery.

HEAVY SNATCH PULL FROM FLOOR

Purpose

To develop strength off the floor and explosive strength during the second pull phase of the snatch.

Action

1. In a standing position, begin with a loaded barbell on the floor approximately a fist width from the shins.

2. Position the heels approximately shoulder-width apart. The feet and knees are slightly turned out.

3. Take a wide overhand or hook grip on the bar. To achieve the ideal starting position, lower the hips, elevate the chest, point the elbows out, direct the eyes slightly upward (more than what is seen in figure 7.7a), and align the head with the spine. The shoulders must remain over the barbell in this set position.

4. Begin the movement by lifting the barbell off the floor by extending the hips and knees while maintaining the barbell close to the shins. The spine remains in a neutral position, with the

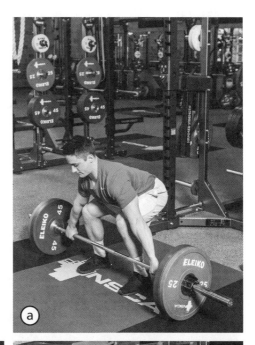

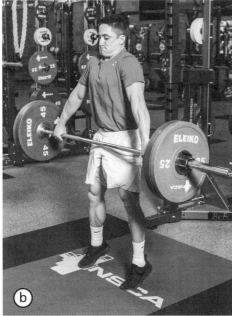

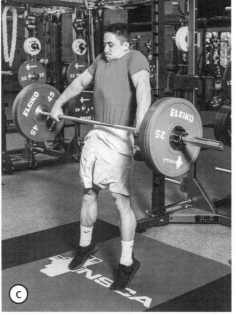

Figure 7.7 Heavy snatch pull from floor *(a)* start position, *(b)* triple extension, and *(c)* shoulder shrug.

(continued)

HEAVY SNATCH PULL FROM FLOOR
(continued)

shoulders over the barbell. Do not let the hips rise before the shoulders rise; the torso-to-floor angle must be kept constant during this phase.

5. As the barbell rises above the knees, begin the second pull by moving the knees under the barbell to allow it to slide up the thighs.

6. Rapidly extend the hips, knees, and ankles (triple extension) while the shoulders remain in line with the barbell and the elbows point out to the sides (figure 7.7*b*).

7. Allow the barbell to slide up the thighs to ensure it remains as close to the body as possible.

8. As the joints of the lower body reach full extension, rapidly shrug the shoulders (figure 7.7*c*).

9. Allow the elbows to naturally flex in a relaxed fashion so the barbell remains close to the body as it rises in the vertical plane.

10. After the bar reaches its maximal height, flex at the knees and the hips to lower the barbell to the starting position on the floor. During this phase, the spine remains in a neutral position, with the shoulders over the barbell.

Note: During this exercise, the arms should remain relaxed and not actively engaged in an attempt to pull the bar up during the top extension phase. Emphasize the triple extension of the lower body, which is immediately followed by the explosive shoulder shrug.

HEAVY SNATCH PULL FROM BLOCKS

Purpose

To develop explosive strength during the second pull phase of the snatch.

Action

1. Using a wide overhand or hook grip, begin with a loaded barbell on a set of lifting blocks. The lifting blocks should be set so that the barbell is positioned just above the knees.
2. At the starting position, the shoulders should be over the barbell, the elbows pointing out, and the head facing forward (figure 7.8a).
3. Rapidly extend the hips, knees, and ankles (triple extension) while the shoulders remain in line with the barbell and the elbows point out to the sides (figure 7.8b).
4. Allow the barbell to slide up the thighs to ensure it remains as close to the body as possible.
5. As the lower body joints reach full extension, rapidly shrug the shoulders.
6. Allow the elbows to naturally flex in a relaxed fashion so that the barbell remains close to the body as it rises in the vertical plane.
7. After the bar reaches its maximal height, flex at the knees and the hips to lower the barbell to the starting position to the blocks. During this phase, the spine remains in a neutral position, with the shoulders over the barbell.

Note: Use blocks of different heights to focus on different phases of the exercise or to make it more specific (e.g., to match the starting position joint angles of a sport-specific movement). In addition, the arms should remain relaxed during this exercise and not actively engaged in an attempt to pull the bar up during the top extension phase.

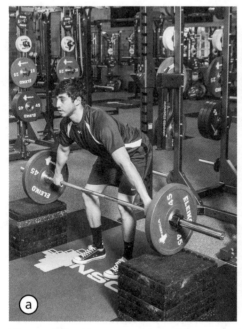 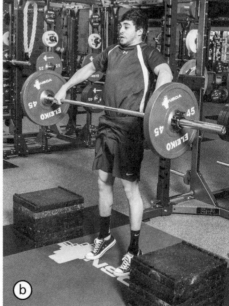

Figure 7.8 Heavy snatch pull from blocks (a) start position and (b) completion of triple extension.

FAST SNATCH PULL FROM FLOOR

Purpose

To develop explosive power from the floor in the vertical plane. This exercise also enables athletes to effectively train the timing and the mechanics of the transition from the explosive second pull to the "pulling under the bar" phase that occurs before moving into the overhead receiving position. Because of the high-speed and complex nature of this exercise, do not perform this movement when fatigued. The correct form must be maintained throughout the execution.

Action

1. To complete the fast snatch pull from floor, refer to points 1-8 of the heavy snatch pull from floor.

2. As the shoulders reach their highest elevation, flex the elbows to forcefully pull the body under the rising barbell as the feet rapidly move into the receiving position. During this phase, the trunk should remain relatively upright; the chest should not lean over the barbell (figure 7.9a-b).

3. Keep the barbell as close to the body as possible during this movement and emphasize attaining a high barbell velocity. Thus, the velocity of the movement greatly dictates the load that should be used.

4. Upon completion of the rapid pulling under phase, flex at the knees and the hips to lower the barbell to the starting position on the floor. During this phase, the spine remains in a neutral position with the shoulders over the barbell.

Note: This exercise is ideal for athletes who are unable to achieve the straight-arm overhead receiving position of the snatch because of injury or mobility issues. However, it is not recommended for those

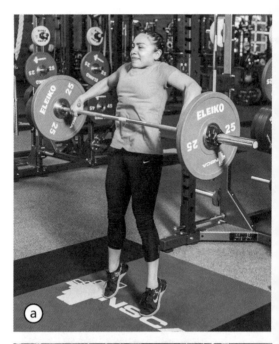

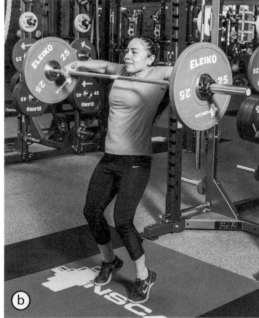

Figure 7.9 Fast snatch pull from floor.

who fail to fully extend during the second pull of the snatch-related exercises because it can reinforce a poor technique habit (e.g., pulling the chest into the barbell). In addition, emphasize the triple extension of the lower body and immediately follow it with an explosive shoulder shrug. Avoid excessive use of the arms during this exercise, and flex the elbows only after completing the lower body triple extension and upper body shrug.

FAST SNATCH PULL FROM BLOCKS

Purpose
To develop explosive power in the vertical plane.

Action

1. Using a wide overhand or a hook grip, begin with a loaded barbell on a set of lifting blocks. Set the height of the lifting blocks so the barbell is positioned just above the level of the knees.

2. At the starting position, the shoulders should be over the barbell, the elbows pointing out, and the head facing forward.

3. Rapidly extend the hips, knees, and ankles (triple extension) while the shoulders remain in line with the barbell and the elbows point out to the sides.

4. To complete the fast snatch pull from blocks (figure 7.10), refer to points 2-3 of the fast snatch pull from floor.

5. Upon completion of the rapid pulling under phase, flex at the knees and the hips to lower the barbell to the starting position on the blocks. During this phase, the spine remains in a neutral position, with the shoulders over the barbell.

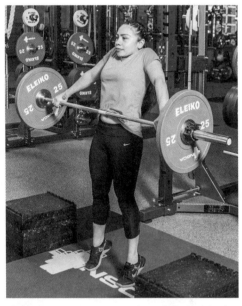

Figure 7.10　Fast snatch pull from blocks.

Note: Because of the high speed and the complex nature of this exercise, don't perform this movement when fatigued. The correct form must be maintained throughout the execution.

SINGLE-ARM DUMBBELL SNATCH

Purpose

To develop explosive power in the vertical plane. This exercise is less technically demanding than the barbell power snatch variations.

Action

1. With the feet positioned approximately shoulder-width apart, straddle a dumbbell. The feet and knees are slightly turned out.

2. Squat at the hips and grasp the dumbbell with a closed, pronated grip. In the starting position, the shoulders should be over the dumbbell, the arm fully extended, and the head facing forward (figure 7.11a). The athlete can also initiate this exercise from a hang position, whereby the dumbbell is lifted to knee level instead of starting from the floor.

3. Begin the upward movement by rapidly extending the hips, knees, and ankles while maintaining the shoulder position over the dumbbell.

4. Allow the dumbbell to rise in the vertical plane while keeping it as close to the thighs as possible.

5. As the lower body joints reach full extension, rapidly shrug the shoulder of the arm that is holding the dumbbell. Place the other hand on the opposite hip or hold the other arm out to the side.

6. When the shoulder reaches its highest elevation, flex the elbow to begin pulling the body under the dumbbell (figure 7.11b). The explosive nature of this phase may cause the feet to lose contact with the floor.

7. Simultaneously flex the hips and knees into a quarter-squat position while forcefully continuing to pull the body under the dumbbell.

8. Once the body is under the dumbbell, catch the weight in the straight-arm overhead receiving position. In the straight-arm overhead receiving position, the dumbbell is positioned over and slightly behind the athlete's ears (figure 7.11c). When viewed from the side, the athlete's ears should not be blocked from view by the arm. Place the other hand on the opposite hip or hold the other arm out to the side for extra balance.

9. Recover to a standing position while maintaining the dumbbell in the straight-arm overhead receiving position.

10. In a controlled fashion, lower the dumbbell to the shoulder, then to the thigh, and finally to the floor. In the hang variation of the dumbbell snatch, the dumbbell does not start on the floor or return to the floor between repetitions.

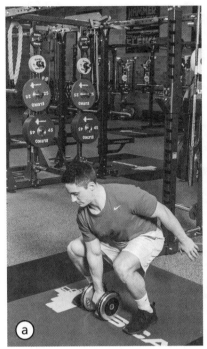
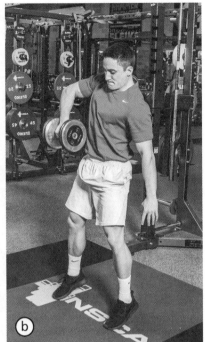
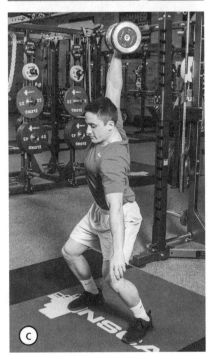

Figure 7.11 Single-arm dumbbell snatch.

POWER CLEAN FROM HANG

Purpose

To develop explosive power in the vertical plane. This exercise is less technically demanding than the power clean from floor.

Action

1. Using a slightly wider than shoulder-width pronated or hook grip, begin by taking hold of a loaded barbell in a lifting rack (or set of blocks) that is set at midthigh height.

2. Position the heels approximately shoulder-width apart, with the feet facing slightly outward.

3. Bend at the knees slightly and flex at the hips to lean the torso forward, allowing the barbell to move down the thighs to a starting position that is just above the knees. At this position, the shoulders should be over the barbell, the elbows pointing out, and the head facing forward (more than what is seen in figure 7.12a) and in line with the spine.

4. Begin the upward movement by rapidly extending the hips, knees, and ankles while maintaining the shoulder position over the barbell.

5. Allow the barbell to slide up the thighs to ensure it remains as close to the body as possible.

6. As the joints of the lower body reach full extension, rapidly shrug the shoulders.

7. When the shoulders reach their highest elevation, flex the elbows to enable the barbell to remain close to the body as it rises in the vertical plane (figure 7.12b). The explosive nature of this phase may cause the feet to lose contact with the floor.

8. Rapidly move the feet and legs into a quarter-squat position while forcefully pulling the body under the barbell.

9. As the body moves under the barbell, rapidly thrust the elbows forward to catch the barbell on the front of the shoulders (figure 7.12c).

10. In the catch position, the torso is nearly erect, the shoulders are slightly in front of the hips and the head remains in a neutral position.

11. Recover to a standing position with the barbell on the front of the shoulders (figure 7.12d).

12. In a controlled fashion, lower the elbows to unrack the barbell from the shoulders, and then slowly lower the barbell to the thighs.

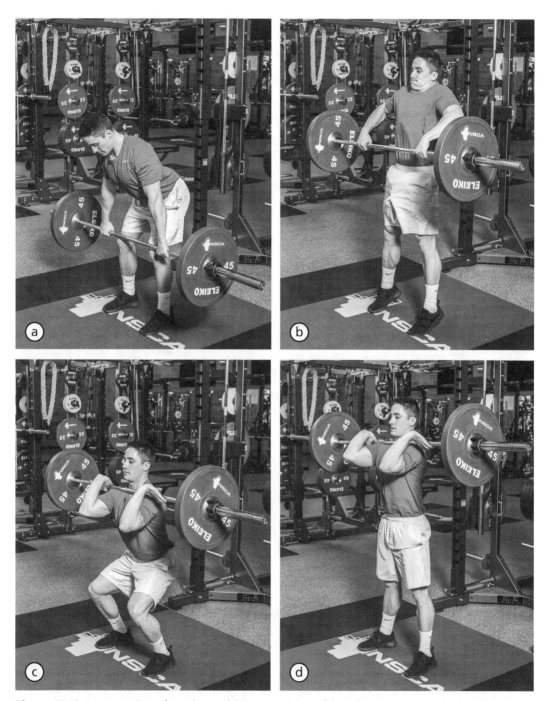

Figure 7.12 Power clean from hang (a) start position, (b) triple extension with shoulder shrug and elbow flex, (c) catch, and (d) recovery.

POWER CLEAN FROM BLOCKS

Purpose
To develop explosive power in the vertical plane by using loads that are typically heavier than those used for the power clean from hang. Conversely, using lighter loads from blocks allows the athlete to focus on the technical aspects of the exercise.

Action

1. Using a slightly wider than shoulder-width pronated or hook grip, begin with a loaded barbell on a set of lifting blocks. Set the height of the lifting blocks so the barbell is positioned just above the knees (figure 7.13a).

2. At the starting position, the shoulders are over the barbell, with the elbows pointing out, the head facing forward (more than what is seen in figure 7.13a).

3. To complete the power clean from blocks (figure 7.13b-c), refer to points 4-11 of the power clean from hang.

4. Upon completion of the recovery phase, lower the elbows to unrack the barbell from the shoulders in a controlled fashion, and slowly lower the barbell to the blocks.

Note: Use blocks of different heights so the athlete can focus on different phases of the exercise.

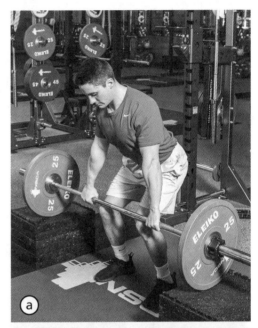

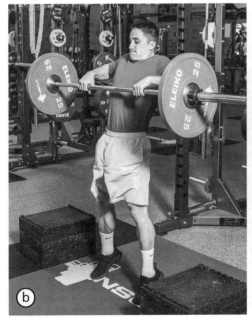
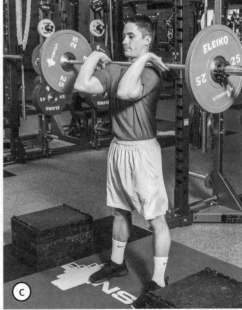

Figure 7.13 Power clean from blocks (a) start position, (b) triple extension with shoulder shrug and elbow flex, and (c) recovery.

POWER CLEAN FROM FLOOR

Purpose

To develop explosive power from the floor in the vertical plane.

Action

1. Begin with a loaded barbell on the floor.

2. Stand with the heels approximately shoulder-width apart and with feet facing forward or slightly outward. Set the barbell approximately a fist width in front of the shins and over the balls of the feet.

3. To achieve an ideal starting position, take a slightly wider than shoulder-width pronated or hook grip, lower the hips, elevate the chest, point the elbows out, and direct the eyes slightly upward. The shoulders must remain over the barbell in this set position while maintaining a neutral back (figure 7.14a).

4. Begin the first pull by extending the knees and hips while maintaining the shoulders over the barbell. Do not let the hips rise before the shoulders rise; the torso-to-floor angle must be kept constant during this phase.

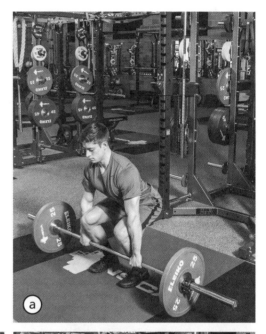

(a)

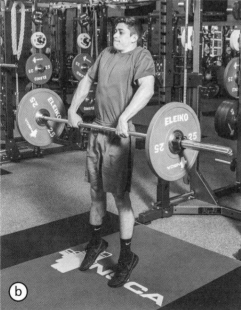

(b)

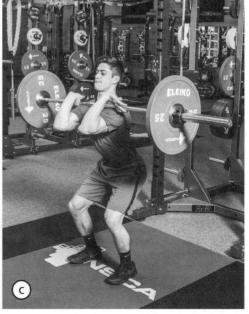

(c)

Figure 7.14 Power clean from floor (a) start position, (b) triple extension with shoulder shrug and start of elbow flex, and (c) catch.

(continued)

POWER CLEAN FROM FLOOR *(continued)*

5. As the barbell rises above the knees, begin the second pull by moving the knees under the barbell to allow it to slide up the thighs.

6. Rapidly extend the hips, knees, and ankles while the shoulders remain in line with the barbell and the elbows point out to the sides.

7. As the lower body joints reach full extension, rapidly shrug the shoulders.

8. When the shoulders reach their highest elevation, flex the elbows to enable the barbell to remain close to the body as it rises in the vertical plane. The explosive nature of this phase may cause the feet to lose contact with the floor (figure 7.14*b*).

9. Rapidly move the feet and legs into a quarter-squat position while forcefully pulling the body under the barbell.

10. As the body moves under the barbell, rapidly thrust the elbows forward to catch the barbell on the front of the shoulders (figure 7.14*c*).

11. In the catch position, the torso is nearly erect, the shoulders are slightly in front of the hips and the head is in a neutral position. (Keep a more closed grip on the bar than what is seen in figure 7.14*c*).

12. Recover to a standing position, with the barbell on the front of the shoulders.

13. In a controlled fashion, lower the elbows to unrack the barbell from the shoulders, and then slowly lower the barbell to the floor.

HEAVY CLEAN PULL FROM FLOOR

Purpose

To develop strength off the floor and explosive strength during the second pull phase of the clean.

Action

1. Begin with a loaded barbell on the floor.

2. Stand with the heels approximately shoulder-width apart, the feet facing forward or slightly outward, and the barbell set approximately a fist width in front of the shins and over the balls of the feet.

3. To achieve an ideal starting position, take a slightly wider than shoulder-width pronated or hook grip, lower the hips, elevate the chest, point the elbows out, and direct the eyes slightly upward. The shoulders must remain over the barbell in this set position while maintaining a neutral back.

4. Begin the first pull by extending the knees and hips while maintaining the shoulders over the barbell (figure 7.15a). Do not let the hips rise before the shoulders; the torso-to-floor angle must be kept constant during this phase.

5. As the barbell rises above the knees, begin the second pull by moving the knees under the barbell to allow it to slide up the thighs.

6. Rapidly extend the hips, knees, and ankles while the shoulders remain in line with the barbell and the elbows point out to the sides.

7. As the lower body joints reach full extension, rapidly shrug the shoulders (figure 7.15b).

8. When the shoulders reach their highest elevation, allow the elbows to flex naturally in a relaxed fashion. This enables the barbell to remain close to the body as the barbell rises in the vertical plane.

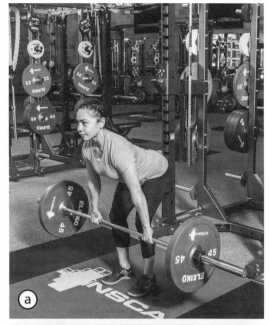

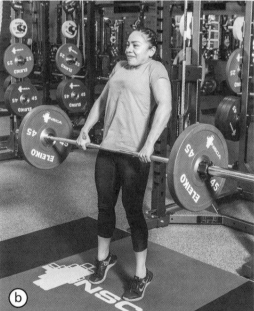

Figure 7.15 Heavy clean pull from floor *(a)* first pull and *(b)* triple extension with shoulder shrug.

9. After the bar reaches its maximal height, flex at the knees and the hips to lower the barbell to the starting position on the floor. During this phase, the spine remains in a neutral position, with the shoulders over the barbell.

Note: During this exercise, keep the arms relaxed and not actively engaged in an attempt to pull the bar up during the top extension phase.

HEAVY CLEAN PULL FROM BLOCKS

Purpose
To develop explosive strength during the second pull phase of the clean.

Action

1. Using a slightly wider than shoulder-width pronated or hook grip, begin with a loaded barbell on a set of lifting blocks. Set the height of the lifting blocks so that the barbell is positioned just above the knees.

2. At the starting position, the shoulders are over the barbell, with the elbows pointing out and the head facing forward.

3. Rapidly extend the hips, knees, and ankles while the shoulders remain in line with the barbell and the elbows point out to the sides.

4. Allow the barbell to slide up the thighs to ensure that it remains as close to the body as possible.

5. As the lower body joints reach full extension, rapidly shrug the shoulders.

6. Allow the elbows to flex naturally in a relaxed fashion to enable the barbell to remain close to the body as the barbell rises in the vertical plane.

7. After the bar reaches its maximal height, flex at the knees and the hips to lower the barbell to the starting position on the blocks. During this phase, the spine remains in a neutral position, with the shoulders over the barbell.

FAST CLEAN PULL FROM FLOOR

Purpose

To develop explosive power from the floor in the vertical plane. This exercise also enables athletes to train the timing and the mechanics of the transition from the explosive second pull to the pulling-under phase that occurs before moving into the barbell-catch position effectively.

Action

1. To complete the fast clean pull from floor, refer to points 1-7 of the heavy clean pull from floor.

2. As the shoulders reach their highest elevation, flex the elbows to forcefully pull the body down as it moves under the barbell and the feet move rapidly into the receiving position (figure 7.16). During this phase, the trunk should remain relatively upright; the chest should not lean over the barbell.

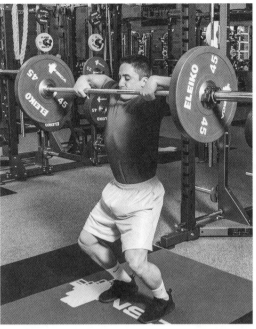

Figure 7.16 Highest bar position of fast clean pull from floor.

3. Keep the barbell as close to the body as possible during this movement, and emphasize an explosive second pull phase.

4. Upon completion of the rapid pulling under phase, flex at the knees and the hips to lower the barbell to the starting position from the floor. During this phase, the spine remains in a neutral position with the shoulders over the barbell.

Note: This exercise is ideal for athletes who are unable to achieve the power clean catch position because of injury or mobility issues. However, it is not recommended for athletes who fail to fully extend during the second pull of the clean-related exercises because it can reinforce a poor technique habit. Although emphasis should be on attaining a high barbell velocity during this exercise, athletes should avoid using the arms excessively during this exercise. The resulting velocity of the movement greatly dictate the loads that can be used. Do not perform this exercise when fatigued because correct technique must be adhered to at all times.

FAST CLEAN PULL FROM BLOCKS

Purpose

To develop explosive power in the vertical plane.

Action

1. Using a slightly wider than shoulder-width overhand or hook grip, begin with a loaded barbell on a set of lifting blocks. Set the height of the lifting blocks so the barbell is just above knee level.

2. At the starting position, the shoulders are over the barbell with the elbows pointing out and the head facing forward (figure 7.17a).

3. Rapidly extend the hips, knees, and ankles (triple extension) while the shoulders remain in line with the barbell and the elbows point out to the sides.

4. To complete the fast clean pull from blocks (figure 7.17b-c), refer to points 2-3 of the fast clean pull from floor.

5. Upon completion of the rapid pulling under phase, flex at the knees and the hips to lower the barbell to the starting position from the blocks. During this phase, the spine remains in a neutral position, with the shoulders over the barbell.

Note: Because of the high speed and complex nature of this exercise, do not perform this movement while fatigued. Correct form must be maintained throughout the execution.

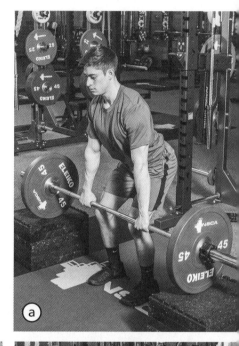

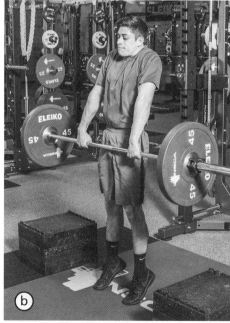

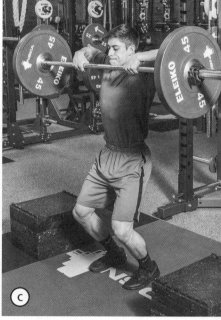

Figure 7.17 Fast clean pull from blocks (a) start position, (b) triple extension with shoulder shrug, and (c) highest bar position.

BARBELL PUSH PRESS

Purpose

To develop overhead strength and explosive power.

Action

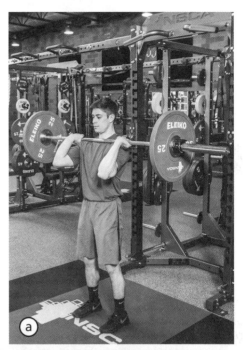

1. Using a slightly wider than shoulder width grip, begin with a loaded barbell set across the shoulders in a fashion similar to the receiving position of a power clean (figure 7.18a).

2. Position the heels hip- to shoulder-width apart, with the feet slightly turned out.

3. While keeping the torso vertical, tuck the chin and initiate the downward movement by flexing the hips and knees. The dip should be relatively shallow, not to exceed a quarter squat (7.18b).

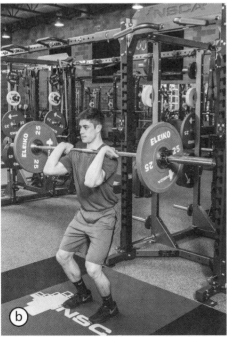

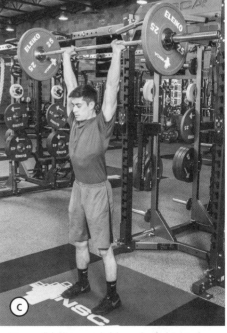

Figure 7.18 Barbell push press (a) start position, (b) dip, and (c) end of drive phase.

(continued)

BARBELL PUSH PRESS *(continued)*

4. At the lowest point of the dip, forcefully drive through the heels by extending the hips, knees, and ankles to raise the barbell in the vertical plane. The timing of the dip into the drive phase should be similar to that of a countermovement jump.

5. Using the momentum created by the leg drive, continue the movement by forcefully pressing the barbell overhead into a fully extended arm position. As the barbell passes past the face, the head is moved from a chin tucked position to a slightly forward position (figure 7.18c).

6. In the straight-arm overhead position, the barbell is slightly over or behind the ears.

7. Lower the barbell by gradually reducing the muscular tension of the arms to allow a controlled descent of the barbell to the shoulders while simultaneously flexing at the hips and knees to cushion the impact.

Note: The body remains in an extended position during the overhead pressing to receiving movement. This differs from the barbell power jerk, which is described next.

BARBELL POWER JERK

Purpose
To develop overhead strength and explosive power.

Action

1. Using a slightly wider than shoulder width grip, begin with a loaded barbell set across the shoulders in a fashion similar to the receiving position of a power clean.

2. Position the heels hip- to shoulder-width apart, with the feet slightly turned out (figure 7.19a).

3. While keeping the torso vertical, tuck the chin and initiate the downward movement by flexing the hips and the knees. The dip should be relatively shallow and should not exceed that of a quarter squat.

4. At the lowest point of the dip, forcefully drive through the heels by extending the hips, knees, and ankles to raise the barbell in the vertical plane. The barbell should remain in a straight vertical path during the jerk dip to jerk drive phases. In addition, the timing of the dip into the drive phase should be similar to that of a countermovement jump (figure 7.19b).

5. Using the momentum created by the leg drive, continue the movement by explosively driving the barbell in the vertical plane (figure 7.19c) as the body is driven underneath the barbell into the straight arm overhead receiving position. As the barbell passes past the face, the head is moved from a chin tucked position to a slightly forward position.

6. In the straight arm overhead receiving position of the power jerk, the barbell is slightly behind the ears and the knees should be flexed to approximately a quarter-squat position (figure 7.19d).

7. Recover to a standing position while maintaining the barbell in the straight-arm overhead receiving position.

8. Lower the barbell by gradually reducing the muscular tension of the arms to allow a controlled decent of the barbell to the shoulders while simultaneously flexing at the hips and knees to cushion the impact.

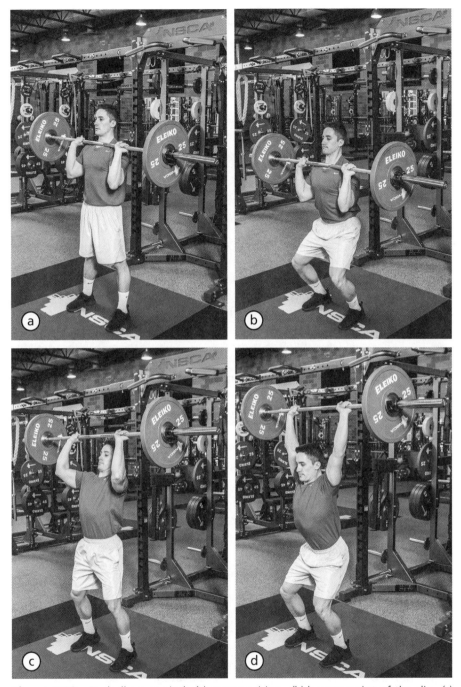

Figure 7.19 Barbell power jerk *(a)* start position, *(b)* lowest point of the dip, *(c)* leg drive, and *(d)* receiving position.

BARBELL SPLIT JERK

Purpose
To develop overhead strength and explosive power.

Action

1. Using a slightly wider than shoulder width grip, begin with a loaded barbell set across the top of the shoulders and the chest.

2. Position the heels approximately shoulder-width apart, with the feet slightly turned out (figure 7.20a).

3. While keeping the torso vertical, tuck the chin and initiate the downward movement by flexing the hips and knees (figure 7.20b). The dip should be relatively shallow and not exceed a quarter squat.

4. At the lowest point of the dip, forcefully drive through the heels by extending the hips, the knees, and the ankles while driving the barbell overhead. As the barbell passes past the face, the head is moved from a chin tucked position to a slightly forward position. The barbell should remain in a straight vertical path during the jerk dip to jerk drive phases. In addition, the timing of the dip into the drive phase should be similar to that of a countermovement jump.

5. As the bar travels upward in the vertical plane, quickly move into the straight-arm overhead receiving position of the split jerk as the bar reaches its highest point. The feet should be positioned approximately shoulder-width apart and evenly split from the starting position in order to achieve a stable lockout position (figure 7.20c).

6. In the receiving or overhead lockout position, the barbell is behind the ears. In addition, the heel of the back foot is raised from the floor and the weight is evenly distributed through both feet.

7. Recover from the split position by returning the front foot to the starting position, followed by the back foot (figure 7.20d).

8. Lower the barbell gradually by reducing the muscular tension of the arms to allow a controlled decent of the barbell to the shoulders while simultaneously flexing at the hips and knees to cushion the impact.

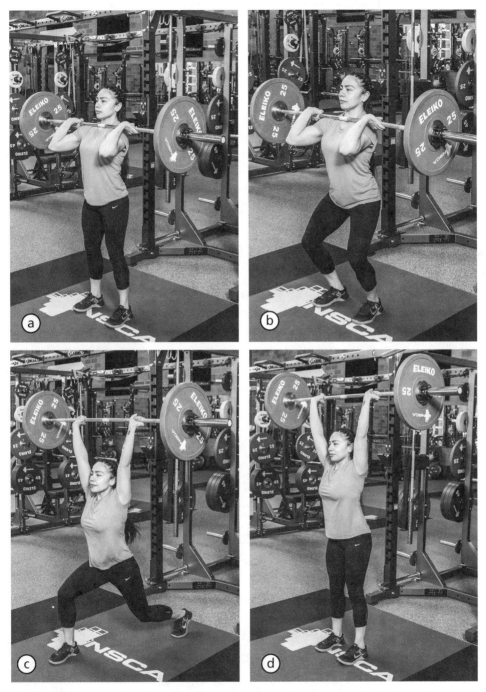

Figure 7.20 Barbell split jerk (a) start position, (b) dip, (c) end of drive phase, and (d) recovery.

DUMBBELL POWER CLEAN TO PUSH PRESS

Purpose

To develop explosive power during a full-body extension and overhead movement.

Action

1. Begin by using a neutral grip to hold a pair of dumbbells. The feet are flat on the floor between hip- to shoulder-width apart and toes pointed slightly outward (figure 7.21a).

2. With a neutral spine, flex at the hips and the knees slightly so the dumbbells are both at a midthigh height and outside of the thighs.

3. Rapidly extend through the hips, knees, and ankles.

4. As the lower body joints reach full extension, rapidly shrug the shoulders.

5. When the shoulders reach their highest point, flex the elbows and receive the dumbbells on the front of the shoulders using a neutral grip. During the catch phase, flex the hips and knees to absorb the impact of the dumbbells (figure 7.21b).

6. Immediately following the dumbbell catch phase, forcefully drive up from the dipped position through the heels to raise the dumbbells in the vertical plane.

7. Using the momentum created by the leg drive, continue the movement by explosively driving the dumbbells overhead (figure 7.21c).

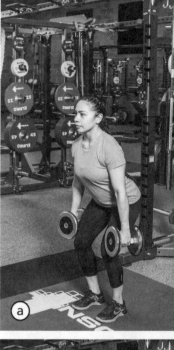

(a)

8. In the straight-arm overhead position, the dumbbells are slightly over or behind the ears with a neutral grip and the legs are fully extended.

9. Lower the dumbbells by gradually reducing the muscular tension of the arms to allow a controlled decent of the dumbbells to the shoulders while simultaneously flexing at the hips and knees to cushion the impact.

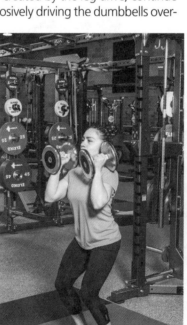

(b)

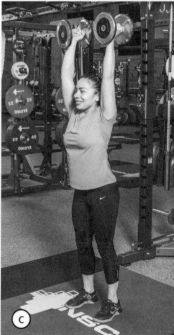

(c)

Figure 7.21 Dumbbell power clean to push press (a) start position (b) catch phase, and (c) leg drive with dumbbells overhead.

CONCLUSION

The total body power exercises described in this chapter are complex whole body movements that have a high degree of transference to many athletic movements such as jumping, sprinting, and change of direction (1, 3, 4, 13, 17). Due to the complex and high-speed demands of these exercises, it is recommended to perform these movements in a non-fatigued state to ensure that correct technique is adhered to while maintaining a high-power focus during the performance of each repetition.

Similarities in set position, lifting, and receiving phases exist between the exercises described in this chapter. Therefore, acquiring an understanding of the key principles of maintaining a neutral spine, keeping the bar close to the body, and developing a strong straight-arm overhead receiving position will aid in the mastery of these movements. In addition, including lifting blocks or performing abbreviated versions of the exercises (e.g. starting from a hang position) enables individuals to focus on different phases of the movement and make the exercise more specific to their needs (e.g., to match the starting position joint angles of a sport-specific movement).

Advanced Power Techniques

Duncan N. French,
PhD, CSCS,*D

In their pursuit of enhanced levels of muscular power, athletes and coaches alike are adopting an ever-increasing number of training strategies that focus on augmenting peak instantaneous power within a given time constant (P_{peak}), or the maximum amount of power output that can be achieved, irrespective of contraction time (P_{max}). This desire reflects the need to express mechanical power in sporting events during discrete muscle actions, where power is often considered a determinant of performance (57, 96). As discussed in previous chapters, central to many current approaches to power training are exercise modalities such as plyometrics, heavy-resistance training, explosive-strength training, and a variety of jumps, throws, strikes, and bounds (23, 77, 95). However, as is apparent with all physical training, prolonged exposure to the same training stimuli can result in an accommodation to the imposed demands and a consequent reduction in the magnitude of physiological adaption (109). Experienced athletes with a long training history who already possess high levels of muscular strength can also demonstrate a reduction in the effectiveness of training regimens that do not offer sufficient variation or overload (17, 18). In both scenarios, when the body either accommodates the training stress, or when an experienced athlete does not exhibit sufficient sensitivity to a specific approach to power training, alternative and more advanced methods must be adopted.

As discussed in previous chapters, mechanical power derives from the force-velocity relationship. All effective power development programs are underpinned by fundamental methods to increase maximal force, maximal contractile velocity, or both physical characteristics concurrently (10, 18, 59). Both traditional approaches to heavy-resistance training (34) and plyometric-type high-velocity training (98) have been shown to change the characteristics of the force–velocity curve (chapter 3). These force–velocity responses are likely the result of morphological changes in the ultrastructure of muscle and tendon or adaptations to the neurological control of muscle activation (19). It is apparent that through fundamental training approaches it is possible to change constituent parts of the force–velocity continuum (e.g., a shift in maximal force), and that such changes lead to consequent alterations in the characteristics of the whole force–velocity curve. In turn, a change in the curvature of the force–velocity relationship can cause an upward shift in the mechanical power product, resulting in a training-induced shift in maximal power output (figure 8.1).

Several studies have demonstrated the benefits of heavy strength training on the expression of P_{max} (4, 17, 94). Other studies have also indicated that high-velocity training (e.g., plyometrics) can improve maximal power output during discrete lower body jumping exercises (32, 98). However, in the applied practice of physical training, where efforts are focused on changing discrete qualities within the force–velocity relationship, there is the risk that reduced training adaptation or even staleness can become apparent (33, 97). Instead, to facilitate continued improvements over time that optimize athletic performance, the athlete's training strategy must be adapted to meet the specific demands of power expression within his or her sport. Therefore, it is conceivable that one mechanical stimulus or one approach to resistance training may not be appropriate for advanced appli-

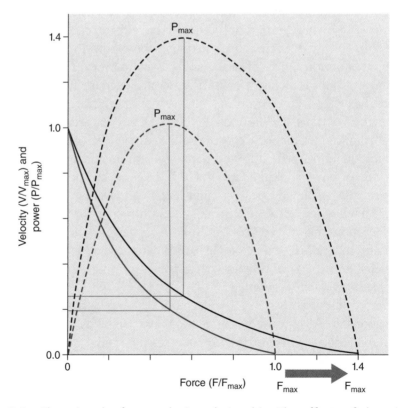

Figure 8.1 Changing the force–velocity relationship. The effects of changing constituent parts of the force–velocity curve (e.g., increased F_{max}) on the associated power output.

cations (37). In such circumstances, by using training methods that introduce more complex stimuli across the whole force–velocity curve, it may be possible to target structural, local, or global factors that regulate power expression. As such, the introduction of advanced power training methods at the correct time and with the appropriate progression may represent the mechanism needed to achieve new gains in muscular power.

TRAINING PHILOSOPHY

When traditional approaches to maximal strength and rate of force development (RFD) training no longer result in the magnitude of physiological or performance adaptation desired, the practitioner must find alternative approaches to muscular power development. Advanced power training methods represent the stimulus required to introduce training variety that ultimately breaks a training plateau or to promote an ongoing increase in performance enhancement through new morphological and neurological adaptation (18). Within any given training regimen are a multitude of opportunities to modulate the characteristics of the training stress in order for it to be considered advanced in its approach. However, it is critical that more complex training methods are brought into the holistic physical development program at the correct time and with the appropriate progression, and that advanced methods are not simply introduced adjunct to fundamental power training methods (i.e., increasing maximal force and maximal velocity). Instead, advanced power training techniques should be considered novel strategies that complement an athlete's individual needs as required. When considering applying advanced methods to affect and augment maximal power output, keep the three Ts in mind: the *tools* used, the *techniques* adopted, and the *tactics* applied. Each of these categories can then be manipulated in order to impart a significant stimulus to the overall training stress (figure 8.2).

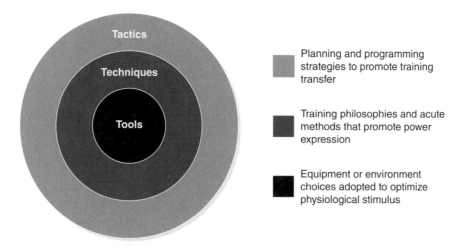

Figure 8.2 Components of advanced power training strategies: tools, techniques, and tactics.

Tools

Tools are the equipment or environmental choices an athlete or coach can adopt in an effort to optimize the training stimulus beyond the methods traditionally used in power training. Strength and conditioning professionals often refer to their "tool box" as the equipment they use to make exercises more challenging or complex. They also use this idea to refer to the way in which they modify equipment to better reflect the biomechanical characteristics desired and the environmental constraints that they place on an athlete in order to challenge force–velocity characteristics. For example, within traditional power training, a decision often considered by strength and conditioning coaches is the execution of Olympic weightlifting variants using either a barbell or dumbbells (chapter 7). Both tools can emphasize the triple extension of the hip, knee, and ankle joints synonymous with peak power outputs (12, 65). However, it is highly likely that the choice of tools will significantly affect biomechanical characteristics, motor unit recruitment, and the nature of the force–velocity relationship that is being accentuated (65).

Techniques

Power training techniques are philosophies and methodologies that can be applied within a given training session to promote muscular power. While all approaches to training might be considered techniques in their own right (e.g., free-weight resistance training vs. plyometric training), our understanding of training science has progressed sufficiently over the past 50 years, such that we can now classify training regimens specifically by the techniques they adopt. For example, eccentric strength training is widely recognized as a training strategy in itself, with a growing body of scientific evidence to support the morphological and performance adaptations that this technique offers (36). Elsewhere, the term *plyometrics* is commonplace. However, within the paradigm of plyometric training, the taxonomy of exercises leads us to further acknowledge the classification of techniques identified as *shock method training* and those simply termed *plyometrics* (102). Consequently, specific training techniques should be considered when planning and programming advanced power training methods (see chapter 3).

Tactics

Finally, the tactics of advanced power training are planning and programming strategies that overarch training methods. They are used within defined phases of training to promote the transfer and realization of power training methods in performance. Programming of advanced training is a central factor in fulfilling the likelihood that a training modality or technique will result in the desired physiological effect. In most instances, the purpose of planning and programming is to manage the fitness–fatigue relationship directly (i.e., overload and recovery) (55, 97). Nowhere should this be more apparent than when performing advanced training methods, during which the optimization of the training stimulus must be apparent because of the rationale that traditional planning and programming methods were failing to impart further beneficial effects, and thus, advanced methods are to be introduced.

METHODS OF ADVANCED POWER TRAINING

The manipulation of acute training variables is at the heart of any advanced training strategy. The manner in which various tools, techniques, and tactics (the three T's) are used by strength and conditioning professionals can profoundly affect performance outcomes. The following sections discuss the three T's in greater detail, and explore which training variables have been demonstrated to have a significant impact during advanced approaches to power training.

Advanced Training Tools

To understand why the use of tools or environmental constraints lend themselves to advanced power training methods, we must first examine force–velocity characteristics. Resistance training methods that use external loads are generally classified as

- ▶ constant resistance, whereby the external load remains unchanged throughout the full range of motion (81);
- ▶ accommodating resistance (also termed *isokinetic resistance*), which allows muscles to contract maximally while the velocity is controlled (70); or
- ▶ variable resistance, which aligns to the force-producing capabilities of the muscle with the mechanical demands throughout a given range of motion (106).

This classification becomes particularly important when exploring torque characteristics (i.e., the relationship between force and joint angle) within the human strength curve (109).

As shown in figure 8.3, the strength curve can be classified into three categories: ascending, descending, and bell shaped (70). Muscle actions with ascending strength curves express strength greatest toward the end of the concentric phase, when joint angles tend to be at their largest (e.g., back squat). Descending strength curves see force optimized in the early portion of the concentric muscle action (e.g., prone row). Single-joint movements such as biceps curls or leg extensions have bell-shaped strength characteristics, whereby force increases to maximum levels in the middle of the range of motion and then is reduced as the range of motion comes to completion (106). By using specific pieces of equipment that affect biomechanical features within a given exercise, it may be possible to directly influence the force-velocity characteristics of respective strength curves and therefore intimately affect the stimulus placed on the muscular and nervous systems. For example, by

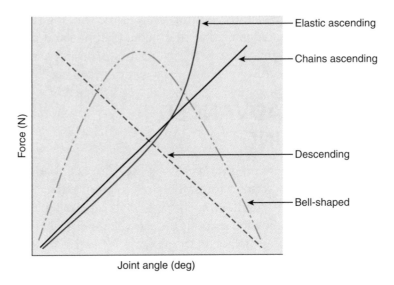

Force (N)

Joint angle (deg)

Elastic ascending

Chains ascending

Descending

Bell-shaped

Figure 8.3 Classification of human strength curves.

applying a variable external resistance to an exercise, it may be possible for a muscle to generate consistently high levels of force throughout the movement, regardless of the nature of the mechanical strength-curve characteristics.

Elastic Bands

The use of elastic resistance in conjunction with free weights is a form of variable resistance training (VRT). As shown in figure 8.3, the viscoelastic properties of an elastic band when it stretches lead to a progressive and sometimes exponential increase in tension that can be applied throughout the range of motion, regardless of joint angle (61). Elastic bands can assist or challenge the human strength curve by varying the tensile load placed on a muscle complex (20, 53, 103). In modern training environments, the use of elastic resistance is becoming commonplace, and research suggests that VRT is a superior method for increasing strength, power (i.e., rate of work per unit of time), and overall electromyography activity when compared to conventional resistance training methods (7, 103).

Training with elastic bands largely challenges ascending strength curves, and the highest resistance is experienced when the elastic is fully stretched. In human biomechanics, this typically corresponds to nearly full extension of the joint and the point of the highest force-producing capabilities (106). This differs from constant resistance or free weights, where the load remains unchanged throughout the range of motion (ROM). This is an important consideration because the mechanical properties of muscle mean there are disadvantages at various positions during a movement task because of the length–tension relationship (i.e., when a joint is in a closed position and the overlap of actin and myosin filaments does not allow for optimal cross-bridge interaction) (109). With the application of elastic resistance to an ascending strength curve, the VRT properties of elastic bands allow for a lighter relative load to be applied at the point when the musculature is at its weakest (in the bottom position of the back squat), and for a greater relative load to be applied at a point in the ROM when muscle is mechanically at its strongest (in the top third of a back squat). In essence, as the movement progresses toward the end of the ROM, the incremental loading associated with elastic bands complements the length-tension relationship by promoting a progressive recruitment of high-threshold motor units (10, 26, 54). As a consequence, the highest motor unit recruitment occurs at the most mechanically advantageous position within a given movement (106). Such increased muscle activation reflects the unique neuromuscular stimulus imparted by the viscoelastic properties of elastic resistance bands (2, 7).

The ability of an athlete to accelerate a load throughout a given range of motion is a critical determinant of power. When training with free weights, the force that is required to move a load is not the same force that is required to keep it moving because of the momentum that the system mass incurs (i.e., the stimulus becomes less with increasing momentum). By using elastic bands, it is possible to affect the amount of momentum achieved within the given ROM of an exercise, such that the athlete must work to accelerate the load for a longer period of time and for a larger portion of the movement. When using advanced power training strategies like this, this is an important consideration. The contractile element of muscle is enhanced by high contraction speeds, and the acceleration of any object is proportional to the force required to move the object but inversely proportional to its mass or inertia. Owing to the way in which elastic bands vary resistance throughout the ROM (i.e., progressively increased tension), their ability to decrease or remove momentum from a system and to promote a greater demand for force would suggest they are a more appropriate modality for developing the force–velocity capabilities required for power expression.

Elastic Bands—Resisted and Assisted?

When performing VRT using elastic bands, coaches and athletes have their choice of methods. The way in which they set up the exercise directly affects the potential to express maximal power output. Used in association with free weights, elastic bands can either resist or assist a given movement pattern. When using elastic resistance, wrap rubber banding around the ends of a barbell and then anchor it to the floor with a heavy weight or the base of a power rack. The force vectors should allow vertical resistance to the floor (61). In such a setup, exercises like the squat, the shoulder press, and the bench press experience the least resistance at the lowest point of bar displacement where there is a mechanical disadvantage. This mitigates the potential effect of sticking points, and allows the bar to be accelerated at a faster rate. With ascending displacement of the bar, the elastic bands stretch and the tension progressively increases; the mechanically strong portion of the exercise is then associated with progressive recruitment of higher-order motor units and a resulting higher P_{peak} (49, 70). The setup for resisted VRT is shown in figure 8.4.

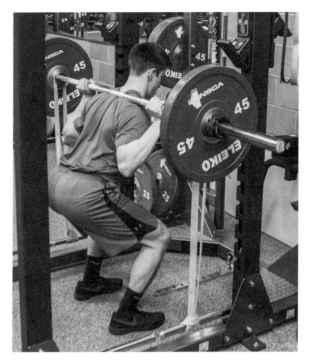

Figure 8.4 Example of a resisted variable resistance training exercise using elastic bands.

In comparison to resisted VRT, assisted training methods are set up with the resistance reversed. In assisted training, the viscoelastic properties of the rubber bands augment the ascent of a bar against gravity. By anchoring the bands at a height (figure 8.5) during bar descent in exercises, such as heavy back squats, the elastic will stretch, reducing the total load at the bottom of the squat. The bands promote rapid movement out of the bottom position. As the athlete rises to return to standing, the magnitude of assistance is reduced throughout the ascent, and the musculature must once again take on more of the force-generating requirements within mechanically advantageous ranges. Assisted VRT methods have been shown to result in greater power and velocity output, with increased shortening rate and neuromuscular system activation reported as potential underlying mechanisms (67, 68, 91).

Programming the use of VRT techniques requires an understanding of the impact that exercise setup has on the nature of the physiological stimulus imposed. When used in a resistive fashion, research suggests that elastic bands both complement the length–tension relationship and promote the progressive recruitment of high-order motor units. Indeed, improvements in RFD have been shown after training with resistive elastic band setups (68, 86, 103). Longer peak-velocity phases, an exploitation of the stretch-shortening cycle (SSC), and an increase in elastic stored energy all were reported. In comparison, assisted VRT exercises may be more desirable during periods of heavy competition, when athlete loads may be

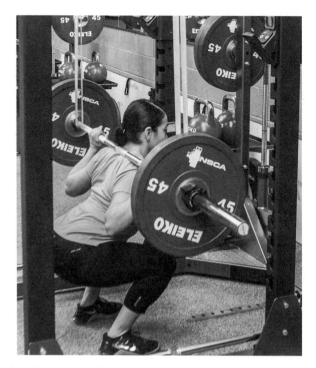

Figure 8.5 Example of an assisted variable resistance training exercise using elastic bands.

compromised by higher levels of fatigue, or during an overspeed training phase, where the speed of movement is the primary training objective (106). Assisting a movement task with the addition of elastic bands allows athletes to explode out of the bottom position of movements, such as the squat or bench press, which in turn increases task specificity, promotes high power outputs, and translates to many ballistic movements found in sport performance, such as jumping and throwing (68, 86). Examples of exercises using bands are outlined in chapters 5 and 6.

Chains

In a similar fashion to the variable load characteristics imparted by the addition of elastic bands, heavy metal chains also represent a valuable method for influencing the force–velocity characteristics of resistance training exercise. The addition of heavy metal chains to alter the force profile of popular resistance exercises such as squats, shoulder presses, and bench presses, has been popular within strength and power training for many years. The popularity of these aids has now spread to the strength and conditioning community, where they are being used for sport performance. As a result, custom-made chains are now commercially available for this specific purpose. Once again, the characteristic feature of this training modality is the ability to vary the resistance directed against a targeted muscle or muscle group over the range of an athletic movement (i.e., VRT) (92).

The use of heavy resistance to develop muscular power is vital because strength is strongly correlated with power output (6). However, using heavy resistance often entails slow lifting velocities (78, 105). This can significantly negate the expression of muscular power (10, 21, 69). Exercises that promote higher contractile velocities throughout the ROM are therefore preferred for the development of P_{peak} within advanced power training methods. As previously discussed, strength curves approximate the torque production capabilities within a given movement. In ascending strength-curve exercises, maximum torque production occurs near the apex of the movement (figure 8.3); therefore, the addition of metal chains that unfurl from the floor as a barbell rises should, in theory, provide increasing resistance to match the changing torque capabilities of the neuromuscular system (60, 71). At the start of the ascending strength curve (e.g., at the bottom of a squat, shoulder press, or bench press) the additional load provided by chains is small, owing to the fact that the chain weight remains largely coiled on the floor. As a consequence, athletes are better able to explode out the bottom portion of an exercise, imparting greater bar velocity and momentum into the system. As the ROM increases and the bar moves farther from the ground, the chains unfurl, adding additional load, but also resulting in augmented muscle stimulation, greater motor unit recruitment, and increased firing frequencies (8, 26). This combination of increased velocity and momentum imparted at the start of the strength curve, added to the progressive increase in muscle activation in the latter portions due to the progressive loading, acts to induce higher P_{peak} outputs within a given exercise (6).

Chains—Optimizing the Stimulus

Increasing amounts of research and anecdotal evidence suggest that the setup of VRT with metal chains is critical in affecting the loading characteristics throughout the ascending strength curve. Traditionally, a linear hanging technique has been adopted, in which chains are directly affixed to either side of a barbell and then are allowed to hang to the ground (74). This linear technique results in a significant portion of the heavy chain hanging as static weight. Only the lower portion of the chain provides variable resistance as it comes into contact with the floor. In contrast, many practitioners are now experimenting with a double-looped or positioning chains approach. Using this method, smaller chains are first affixed to the barbell. Then, heavier chains are looped through the smaller ones. Neelly et al. (74) report that when using the double-looped method, 80%-90% of the chain weight load experienced at the top of a back squat is completely unloaded at the bottom of the squat. This means that during the ascent of the bar, 80%-90% of the chain weight is progressively added to the total system load as the chain unfurls from the floor. In contrast, in the linear hanging method, only 35%-45% of the total chain weight is added to the ascending strength curve; the rest of the chain simply hangs as static weight (74). These findings suggest a nearly twofold difference in the amount of variable resistance provided between the double-looped and the linear hung method and as such, strength and conditioning professionals should consider the importance of VRT exercise setup.

Bands or Chains?

A host of research has highlighted the differences between elastic bands and chains, with elastic bands exhibiting a curvilinear tension-deformation relationship and chains exhibiting a linear mass-displacement relationship (6, 70, 71, 92, 103). The characteristics of these length–tension relationships should guide strength and conditioning practitioners in their decisions about advanced power training methodology. For example, muscle actions in which force characteristics are accumulative toward the end of a movement (e.g., a punch in boxing, vertical jump in basketball) might be better suited to elastic band VRT, and sporting actions requiring a consistent application of force (e.g., scrummaging in rugby, block start in sprinting) might be better suited to chain VRT. By choosing the appropriate methodology, it is likely that the intermuscular specificity will more closely resemble the force–velocity characteristics experienced during the discrete sport performance.

While a recent meta-analysis by Soria-Gila et al. (92) has reported the comparative effects of VRT using bands or chains on maximal strength, a similar comprehensive analysis of maximal power adaptations has not been conducted. This makes comparing the benefits of each of these VRT methods difficult. However, what is apparent is that VRT is not recommended for untrained subjects because the increases in force characteristics that this population makes using such methods of training are similar to the gains experienced with traditional free-weight training alone (17). This supports the use of VRT as an advanced power training method, with trained athletes experiencing improved force–velocity characteristics above that of traditional training (2, 6, 92).

ADVANCED POWER TRAINING TECHNIQUES

Advanced power training techniques are used in the day-to-day training environment and emphasize particular biomotor characteristics associated with the expression of high power outputs. When using advanced approaches to training, consider the classification of training modalities relevant to the techniques adopted; doing so can bring clarity and focus to the holistic planning process. By focusing training on the implementation of specific training techniques, it is possible to better understand the impact that a particular training intervention has on maximal power output, and how it ultimately affects performance outcomes.

Ballistic Training

In simple terms, what differentiates exercises that develop strength from exercises that develop power is whether the performance of the exercise entails acceleration of a load throughout the majority of the ROM; this results in faster movement speeds and thus higher power outputs (3, 77). Power exercises are characterized by high-velocity movements that accelerate the athlete's body or an object throughout the ROM with a limited braking phase and little, if any, slowing of contractile velocity. A comprehension of full acceleration and movement speed is important within the paradigm of power training because athletes are often instructed to move a load as fast as possible, often using lighter relative loads in order to be powerful. However, the problem with conventional resistance training techniques is that even when using lighter loads, power decreases in the final half of a repetition in order for the athlete to decelerate the bar and for the bar to achieve zero velocity (77). This is so an athlete can maintain his or her grip on the bar and bring the bar to a static position under control at the end of the ROM. When resistance exercises are performed in this traditional fashion, Elliot et al. (28) reported that the deceleration of a bar accounts for 24% of the movement with a heavy weight and 52% of the movement with a light weight. Furthermore, this deceleration phase is accompanied by a significant reduction in electromyogram (EMG) activity of the primary agonist muscles recruited in the movement (28, 77). Therefore, in any one movement, a quarter to half of the full ROM is actually spent slowing rather than trying to generate explosive contractile characteristics.

Ballistic training refers to when an athlete attempts to accelerate a weight throughout the full ROM of an exercise, which often results in the weight being released or moving freely into space with momentum. Examples of ballistic exercises are shown in table 8.1 and are described in more detail in chapters 5 and 6. Investigating the ballistic bench throw exercise, Newton et al. (77) report that ballistic movements produce significantly higher outputs for average velocity, peak velocity, average force, and, most important, average power, and peak power than traditional methods. Furthermore, during ballistic training, the bar can be accelerated for up to 96% of the movement range, causing greater peak bar velocities and allowing the muscles to produce tension over a significantly greater period of the total concentric phase. Even when performed under heavier loading conditions (e.g., >60% of 1RM) which would severely limit an athlete's ability to release a weight into free space, the intent to propel a load into the air is superior to traditional resistance training methods for the development of maximal power output (16).

Training to maximize power output for advanced training should entail not only slower heavy-resistance exercises for strength development, but it should also involve high-velocity ballistic exercises in which acceleration of an external load is promoted throughout the entire ROM (3, 75). The most common ballistic

Table 8.1 Classification of Strength-Based Exercises and Equivalent Ballistic Exercise (Power) Variations

Strength exercise	Ballistic variation (power)
Squat	Jump squat
Split squat	Alternating lunge jump
Single-leg squat	Single-leg hop
Deadlift	Power clean, snatch, fast clean pull
Bench press	Bench throw
Seated row	Bench pull
Military press	Push jerk
Push-up	Clap push-up

exercises used in athletic performance training are the loaded countermovement jump (CMJ) for the lower body (e.g., jump squat), and the Smith machine bench throw for the upper body (3, 5, 76, 77). Plyometrics (32) and Olympic weightlifting (48) can also be considered ballistic in nature because they too encourage full acceleration. In the case of weightlifting, bar velocities are affected only by gravity. For example, the slow contractile velocities involved in powerlifting (back squat, deadlift, and bench press) have been shown to generate approximately 12 W/kg of body weight in elite weightlifters (39). In comparison, the second pull of Olympic weightlifting movements, such as the snatch or the clean, produce on average 52 W/kg of body weight in the same population of athletes (39). These data are largely a consequence of the ballistic nature of Olympic weightlifting movements, where athletes try to accelerate a barbell for up to 96% of the movement (e.g., clean, snatch) in an attempt to impart momentum into the bar before dropping under it as it continues to rise in free space, thus allowing the athletes to move into the catch, or receiving, position (100) (see also chapter 7).

The mean velocities of ballistic movements are greater than those of nonballistic movements because there is no deceleration or braking phase in ballistic movements. This is supported by Frost et al. (37), who observed that significantly higher power measures are found during ballistic exercises, largely as a result of their higher mean velocity. Lake et al. (62), however, challenged the superiority of lower body ballistic exercises for power development. Studying moderately well-trained men, the authors suggest that while higher mean velocity (14% greater) is seen in ballistic exercise, there is no difference between ballistic and traditional training methods when comparing the RFD during an exercise. Data such as these continue to challenge our understanding of the kinematics related to ballistic training methods. What is apparent, however, is that consideration must be given to the manner in which ballistic exercises are interpreted. If instantaneous P_{peak} is recorded, it is likely that the impact of ballistic exercise on power characteristics may be equivocal between moderately trained and well-trained people. If, however, P_{max} is a more important variable to pursue, Frost et al. (37) suggest this may better differentiate well-trained athletes when compared to moderately trained people. Such comparisons potentially lead us to conclude that ballistic training methods are better suited to advanced athletes who already possess high levels of muscular strength and require substantial complexity and variation within their training program in order to augment the desired adaptation in force–velocity characteristics.

Velocity-Based Training

When developing advanced training strategies, athletes and coaches should consider the time available within discrete motor skills in which to produce peak force. While the majority of weight room–based strength training exercises take several seconds to complete a single repetition, rarely in sport is time sufficient within athletic movements to achieve maximal force, with instantaneous peak force (F_{peak}) instead largely occurring between 0.101 s and 0.300 s (table 8.2). Therefore,

Table 8.2. Time Constraints of Explosive Force Production Within Discrete Sporting Movements

Sport and motion	Time to peak force	Reference
Sprint running	0.101 (males) 0.108 (females)	Mero and Komi (72)
Long jump	0.105-0.125 (males)	Zatsiorsky (108)
High jump	0.15-0.23 (males) 0.14 (females)	Dapena (22)
Platform diving	1.33 (standing takeoff) 0.15 (running dive)	Miller (73)
Ski jumping	0.25-0.30	Komi and Virmavirta (58)
Shot putting delivery	0.22-0.27 (male)	Lanka (63)

velocity specificity should be a central consideration when training to develop muscular power, with the physiological adaptations being velocity dependent (54, 69) and the greatest adaptations occurring at or near the training velocities (80). Owing to recent technological advancements and improved diagnostic techniques, the opportunity to gain insight into the force–velocity characteristics of discrete exercises and movement patterns has increased. As a result, velocity-based training (VBT) is becoming a popular way to determine optimal resistance training loads through real-time biometric feedback that reports repetition-to-repetition performance. More specifically, monitoring repetition velocity helps to dictate the speed at which a training exercise should be performed. When combined with moderate to high external loads, the intent to move at high speeds can enhance the relative and absolute power output in the concentric phase of muscle actions (84).

Why Velocity-Based Training?

Historically, strength and conditioning practitioners have prescribed resistance training loads based on a percentage of a previously determined 1RM. Exercises are performed and progress at various submaximal intensities (e.g., loaded CMJ at 40% of 1RM back squat). While sound in principle, using % 1RM can be challenging from a practical perspective. Unless daily 1RMs are established, training at a specific % 1RM may be flawed. Testing for 1RM can take a significant amount of time, making it logistically difficult to schedule into a program regularly. Furthermore, the accuracy of 1RM testing is affected by daily levels of motivation. Add to this the potential change over time in 1RM performance that may occur as a consequence of training, and accurately gaining a measure of true max can be challenging at best. In comparison, VBT relies on rep-to-rep instantaneous feedback relating to the velocity of a barbell or weight. This allows variation in training loads across a training phase so long as the athlete consistently maintains a specified bar speed threshold. This bar velocity, or velocity-based training, can then be related to the stimulus for a specific strength quality (figure 8.6).

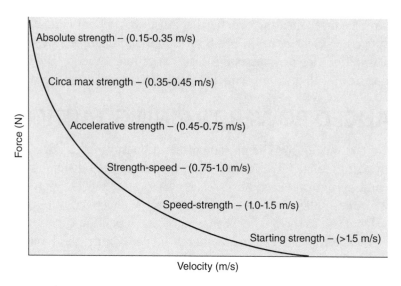

Figure 8.6 labels (within figure):
- Absolute strength – (0.15-0.35 m/s)
- Circa max strength – (0.35-0.45 m/s)
- Accelerative strength – (0.45-0.75 m/s)
- Strength-speed – (0.75-1.0 m/s)
- Speed-strength – (1.0-1.5 m/s)
- Starting strength – (>1.5 m/s)
- Force (N)
- Velocity (m/s)

Figure 8.6 Velocity-based training curve illustrating the relationship between specific strength qualities and associated bar velocities during resistance training.

A nearly perfect linear relationship has been reported between % 1RM and the corresponding bar velocity (41). Monitoring the velocity of a movement can therefore be used to periodize training and promote desired neuromuscular adaptations specific to power expression. By objectively measuring bar velocity to implement neuromuscular overload rather than using the traditional change in % 1RM load, it is possible to use the speed of a movement as the mechanism to challenge the physiological adaptations that underpin power expression. For example, when examining the strength continuum (figure 8.6), 40%-60% 1RM is representative of both strength-speed and speed-strength qualities, with velocities between 0.75-1.50 m/s (21). While both of these traits require the expression of high levels of muscular power, they are in fact different and can easily be discerned by velocity, a major advantage of VBT. Strength-speed is defined as moving a moderately heavy weight as fast as possible (i.e., moderate loads at moderate velocities), and has been shown to exist at 0.75-1.00 m/s (50, 52). In comparison, speed-strength exercises include velocities ranging from 1.0-1.5 m/s. They are best described as speed in the conditions of strength, or speed prioritized over strength (50, 52), thus allowing lighter loads to be moved at high velocities.

Indeed, the value of velocity-based resistance training is supported by several research studies (9, 84, 85). For example, when investigating the effects of instantaneous performance feedback (peak velocity) after each repetition of squat jump exercises over 6 weeks in professional rugby players, Randell et al. (85) demonstrated improvements in the performance of sport-specific tests that suggest greater adaptation and larger training effects occur using VBT feedback (e.g., 0.9%-4.6% improvement with VBT vs. 0.3%-2.8% without). By providing velocity-based targets and thresholds during training, these researchers proposed that the probability of in-the-action feedback creating beneficial change was 45% for vertical jump, 65% for 10 m sprints, 49% for 20 m sprints, 83% for horizontal jump, and 99% for 30 m sprints. These findings demonstrate the potential magnitude to which velocity-based indices can influence subsequent sport-specific performance standards.

ADVANCED POWER TRAINING TACTICS

The ability to stimulate specific physiological and performance adaptations optimally is in part predicted by the ability to vary the training demands and induce novel stimuli at appropriate times (97). Power production is a consequence of efficient neuromuscular processes, and therefore the effectiveness of power training is largely related to the quality with which each repetition is performed or the magnitude of fatigue-related remnants that influence contractile characteristics or both. Baker and Newton (5) suggest both that it is important to avoid fatigue when trying to maximize power output, and that performing a low number of repetitions with an appropriate rest interval optimizes power training. When developing an approach to optimize muscular power production, the ability to introduce appropriate training variation in a logical and systematic fashion that complements the development of specific physiological attributes is essential (44). When implementing a periodized advanced power training program, one can introduce variation at many levels, including the manipulation of the overall training load, the number of sets and repetitions, the number of exercises, the exercise order, the focus of the training block, and the rest interval between sets (see chapter 3). Therefore, strength and conditioning professionals must appropriately consider the planning and programming tactics they can implement if they are to significantly affect adaptive processes consequent to training.

Cluster-Set Training

To promote the development of muscular maximal power output, repetitions of a given exercise should achieve ≥90% of maximal power output and velocity for the stimulus to be considered beneficial (33). Achieving such high-intensity thresholds becomes critical, and the manner in which exercises are prescribed becomes fundamental in determining their effectiveness. In a classical sense, training sets normally comprise a series of 3-20 repetitions performed in a continuous fashion. When examining this traditional set configuration, however, it is apparent that bar velocity, peak power output, and bar displacement all decrease with each subsequent repetition in a set, largely as a result of accumulating fatigue (38, 45). One must introduce alternative methods in order to maintain the performance standard for each repetition.

The ability to perform power training in a nonfatigued state, whereby a more optimal training stimulus can enhance neural adaptations, is a central philosophy behind the use of cluster-set training (see chapter 3). Strength and conditioning professionals can modify the structure of a cluster set to target specific physiological and performance characteristics. Specifically, in advanced power training regimens, cluster sets provided an important tactic that optimizes the development of muscular force–velocity capabilities.

Postactivation Potentiation

The performance characteristics of skeletal muscle are transient in nature and can be intimately affected by contractile history (88). French et al. (35) report that following heavy loading, the strength and power characteristics of subsequent muscle actions can be temporarily improved under the influence of an increased excitability of the central nervous system. This increased neural excitation is the result of an acute physiological adjustment that has been referred to as postactivation potentiation (PAP) (47, 99). The PAP phenomenon is widely accepted in strength and conditioning literature. The underlying premise is that prior heavy loading can maximize subsequent explosive activity by inducing a high degree of neural stimulation that results in greater motor unit recruitment and high-frequency rate coding. The application of this premise is commonplace as an advanced training method. The underlying mechanisms associated with improved contractile properties are attributed to the phosphorylation of myosin regulatory light chains, which make the contractile proteins of actin and myosin in muscle fibers more sensitive to calcium. Calcium is a central regulator of neural activity, meaning that each nervous signal sent within a motor unit has a direct impact on a muscle's capacity to contract (47, 79). Increased recruitment of larger fast-twitch motor units has also been proposed as a potential determining factor for the enhanced force production (99). If used effectively, PAP can be implemented into a power-training program for the purpose of enhancing the magnitude of the training stimulus of other explosive movements (24, 87). Indeed, research suggests that the effects of PAP are observed as a positive bias for subsequent muscle actions (43), with the magnitude and decay characteristics of the performance bias intimately related to the intensity and duration of any conditioning precontractions (90).

Preconditioning activities, while enhancing PAP, also fatigue skeletal muscle (14, 99). The balance between PAP and fatigue and their effects on subsequent explosive contractions is therefore a delicate one. The optimal window for affecting performance depends on the amplitude and the rate of decay of both PAP and fatigue. Peak PAP occurs immediately following a preconditioning activity, although this is unlikely to be the time at which peak performance is evident, because it is also the time of peak fatigue. Similarly, the greater the time between conditioning activity and subsequent performance, the greater the recovery from fatigue and the greater the decrement in PAP (51).

An optimal recovery time is required to realize PAP and diminish fatigue. Gullich and Schmidtbleicher (43) and Gilbert et al. (40) reported no change in isometric RFD immediately following conditioning contractions; however, following sufficient recovery of 4.5-12.5 min and up to 15 min, increases of 10%-24% were observed respectively. In a similar fashion, Kilduff et al. (56) demonstrated a 7%-8% increase in countermovement jump peak power 8-12 min following conditioning contractions, while Chatzopoulos et al. (13) showed 30 m sprint performance increased 2%-3% 5 min afterward. These results differ from French et al. (35), who did not use a recovery period, but still observed significant increases in both drop-jump height and acceleration impulse knee-extension peak torque immediately following three sets of 3 s isometric maximum voluntary contractions. Elsewhere, Chiu et al. (15) were unable to detect significant improvement in the peak power of three CMJs or three loaded squat jumps at 40% 1RM, even when performed after a recovery period of 5, 6, and 7 min following back squats at 90% 1RM.

An important consideration for advanced power training techniques is the magnitude of individual PAP responses and how they are influenced by characteristics of individual athletes, including muscular strength, fiber-type distribution, training history, and power-strength ratios. In elite rugby players already possessing high levels of muscular strength and a long training history, Kilduff et al. (56) reported a positive correlation between stronger athletes (absolute and relative) and peak power output during a CMJ test 12 min after they each performed potentiating 3RM back squats. Gourgoulis et al. (42) indicate that individual strength levels are important when trying to maximize the PAP effect, reporting a 4% increase in CMJ in stronger participants able to squat >160 kg compared to an increase of only 0.4% in weaker athletes squatting <160 kg. Such strength-based comparisons are supported by cellular-level characteristics, with people exhibiting predominantly fast-twitch muscle fibers (Type II) able to elicit a greater PAP response than people with high numbers of slow-twitch (Type I) fibers (46). However, people with predominantly Type II fibers also elicited the greatest fatigue response following conditioning contractions (46), highlighting the importance of administering PAP protocols. An athlete's training history is also an important consideration for the expression of PAP. When comparing athletes who were training to compete in sports at a national or international level to those who undertook recreational resistance training, Chiu et al. (15) found significant differences in the nature of the PAP–fatigue relationship. Following 5 sets of 1 repetition of back squats at 90% 1RM and 5-7 min of subsequent recovery, the advanced training group exhibited a 1%-3% increment in CMJ and SJ performance; whereas, the recreational trainers experienced a 1%-4% reduction in performance.

The opportunity to use the physiological characteristics associated with PAP is an attractive consideration for athletes and coaches seeking to enhance the mechanical power stimulus associated with explosive training modalities. However, because of the number of influencing factors, it can be challenging to effectively exploit PAP (89). Inconsistent results from research further challenge the clarity with which this training methodology should be implemented. As illustrated earlier, advanced athletes who train at higher levels and have greater muscular strength, a greater fast-twitch fiber distribution, and a lower power-strength ratio are likely to benefit from the inclusion of PAP techniques in their training program. Coaches and athletes can implement PAP techniques both in training (see sections on complex and contrast training later in this chapter) and immediately before a competition or sporting skill that requires high levels of muscular power expression (e.g., before jump performance or push starts in the bobsled) (see chapters 9 and 10 for examples). With results showing the potential for a 2%-10% increase in performance following PAP strategies, the value of these methods certainly warrants acknowledgement for advanced performers. To promote the expression of PAP, the following recommendations are given:

▶ Effective application of PAP requires determining the optimal application for each athlete before using it within competition environments or heavy training phases.

▶ Maximal contractions and heavy external loads appear to offer the best opportunity to elicit PAP, and while no definitive optimal load is evident, loads should directly recruit the Type II muscle fibers, and thus will need to be ≥90% 1RM.

▶ Optimal rest periods vary among athletes and depend on the interaction between potentiation and fatigue. Practitioners and athletes should determine the appropriate rates of recovery following conditioning activity for each athlete.

▶ Only experienced athletes with an extensive training history should use PAP strategies for precompetition priming or as a training stimulus.

▶ Contrasting loads that provide a strength–power potentiating complex within a training regimen may be an effective way to use PAP when the expression of muscular power is a critical outcome of the training phase.

Complex Training

The neuromuscular phenomenon of postactivation potentiation can be harnessed in a training environment with the objective of intensifying a neuromuscular stimulus. Complex training or use of strength–power potentiation complexes is an advanced programming strategy that involves alternating biomechanically similar high-load weight training exercises with plyometric-type exercises (83), with the completion of all the heavy sets first followed by lighter power and plyometric exercises. Complex training was first presented by Verkhoshansky and Tatyan (101), who postulated that resistance exercise will have a performance-enhancing effect (i.e., potentiating) on plyometric activity by increasing power output and stretch-shortening cycle efficiency. More recently, Ebben and Watts described the effectiveness of combining strength training and plyometric activities and presented strategies for including both of these divergent strength characteristics in the same workout session (27). For example, a complex training strategy may involve 3 × 5 heavy back squats at 87.5% 1RM followed by 3 × 6 jump squats at body weight.

The fashion in which complex training sets are structured reflects the mechanism by which potentiation of the neuromuscular system augments explosive muscle actions following preconditioning contractile activity. Indeed, several studies have demonstrated how enhanced motor performance during plyometric training can occur when combined with traditional weight training (1, 31, 64). Maio Alves et al. (66) have demonstrated such training responses after 6 weeks of complex training in elite youth soccer players, with increased performances found in 5 m (7%-9.2%) and 15 m (3.1%-6.2%) sprint times as well as squat jump height (9.6%-12.6%). Like all programming strategies that aim to augment PAP responses, complex training program design must always consider important variables such as exercise selection, load, and rest between working sets (25).

Complex training is not a new approach to power training. Early studies of strength–power potentiating complexes reported them to be effective for both the upper (29) and lower body (82) and to be more effective in men than women (82). Both the prerequisite strength and the intensity of the load used in the resistance training portion of the complex appear to be important regulators in eliciting the complex training effect during subsequent plyometric conditions (107). While more research is required, some studies have reported that children and female athletes show inconclusive responses to complex training when compared to basic strength training programs (30, 110, 82). This lack of significant difference between methods is likely a reflection of the fact that specific population groups that lack the prerequisite strength necessary will likely experience limited benefit from the effects that complex training (i.e., PAP) might offer (15, 27). In contrast, in well-trained collegiate NCAA Division I football players who were engaged in a periodized resistance training program for 1-5 years, complex training methods have been found to promote significantly more improvement in vertical jump performance than traditional training methods (11). Similar changes in jumping ability following complex training stimuli have been reported elsewhere within the literature (66, 107).

Contrast Training

Similar to complex training, contrast training is also a planning and programming strategy that aims to accentuate the neuromuscular characteristics associated with PAP. Unlike complex training, contrast training uses sets of biomechanically similar movements, but with very different loads in order to create a stark and purposeful divergence in contractile velocities. Complex training uses of multiple sets, or complexes, of heavy-resistance exercise followed by several sets of plyometric exercise. Contrast training instead relies on alternating heavy and light exercises; a set of high-velocity muscle actions follows each set of heavier high-force exercises (83). In principle, this approach alternates sets of heavy-resistance loads with sets of plyometric exercise, for example, using 1 × 5 back squats at 87% 1RM followed by 1 × 6 jump squats at 30% 1RM for 3 sets. Like complex training, contrast training adopts heavy resistances because they appear to create a greater activation and preparation for ensuing maximal effort in subsequent explosive movements (87, 99, 107).

While the most effective methodology for optimizing PAP in both complex and contrast training regimens remains to be fully elucidated, researchers and practitioners generally agree that combining high-resistance loads with lighter, high-velocity movements produces optimal gains in power output. In comparing the respective benefits of both these approaches, Rajamohan et al. (83) showed better effects in contrast-trained athletes in both strength and power parameters when compared to complex-trained athletes after 12 weeks of training. Changes in explosive power was interpreted as gains in both vertical and horizontal jump performances, with contrast training indicating a 3.17% and 5.9% increase over complex training methods, respectively.

While contrast training has traditionally involved very heavy loads followed by lighter loads or body-weight exercise, Sotiropoulos et al. (93) recently investigated using a contrast training protocol that adopted a predetermined load that maximized mechanical power output in resisted jump squats (P_{max}), a 70% P_{max} load, and a 130% P_{max} load. These data were then compared to repeated vertical jumps at body weight. These authors reported that the load that maximizes external mechanical-power output compared with a heavier or a lighter load, using the jump squat, is not more effective for increasing jumping performance afterward. These data perhaps reinforce that the intensity of the loading strategy used for any preconditioning activity that is trying to harness the neuromuscular characteristics of PAP is critical in determining a beneficial outcome. In exploring data such as these, it is apparent that science has yet to fully elucidate the exact mechanisms that support PAP during contrast training methods. While research continues to answer this complex question, applied practitioners continue to engage with the anecdotal benefits to performance observed during advanced training strategies.

IMPLEMENTING ADVANCED TRAINING METHODS

As discussed within this and previous chapters, the ability to generate maximal muscular power is multifaceted, with many contributing factors affecting power expression (19). The manner in which coaches and athletes impart a training overload on the neuromuscular system regulates the development of muscular power. , While power training strategies have been shown to effectively improve muscular power in some people, they have not in others (18, 19). Therefore, it is critical that the implementation of advanced training methods is conducted in a fashion that will meet the specific needs of the individual athlete.

In the early stages of power training, it is likely that changes in the force–velocity relationship are the consequence of gains in basic muscular strength. However, with advancing years of training history, athletes can exploit the gained adaptations in neuromuscular synchronization and increased Type IIa fibers to further enhance power expression through training methods that harness these new physiological attributes. Heavy strength training improves maximal power output in relatively untrained or weak people (1, 104, 105), but not in stronger, more experienced athletes (76, 104). Instead, stronger athletes who possess greater levels of basic strength appear to best develop ongoing muscular power expression by increasing complexity in their training stimulus, specifically the addition of velocity-based exercises (3). Indeed, while continuing to maintain high levels of maximal strength, advanced athletes should use exercises that promote the maximal shortening properties of muscle (i.e., maximal velocity) in an effort to alter the characteristics of the neuromuscular system. In turn, this will change the profile of the force-velocity curve and affect the muscular power product. The inclusion of principles of advanced power training into the training program of well-trained athletes has the capacity to promote ongoing gains in maximal power output.

CONCLUSION

Throughout this chapter we have presented the tools, techniques, and tactics one can implement into advanced training programs in an effort to develop muscular power. By understanding human strength curves, one can introduce advanced power training methods in a way that affects muscular force production within given exercises. The strength and conditioning professional's equipment choices can significantly affect how the neuromuscular system is required to express muscular power. Beyond that, by comprehending the importance that full acceleration throughout the ROM has on power output, ballistic exercises then offer a unique challenge to advanced athletes. During this process, it is prudent to cover a wide range of loading schemes in an effort to challenge the expression of instantaneous P_{peak} rather than focusing on an athlete's maximal power output. In doing so, the ever-changing resistances and velocities will better reflect the power expression characteristics experienced in sporting competition. Modulating training program structures through distinct changes in exercise prescription (e.g., cluster sets, complex training) may be an efficient means to enhance power output by managing fatigue or by promoting physiological phenomena that optimize power output (i.e., postactivation potentiation) or both. At minimum, programming strategies provide clarity in the organizational approach to power training that will help an athlete understand how the neuromuscular system should be challenged in order to challenge optimal thresholds of muscular power development. Chapters 9 and 10 present examples of these programming strategies.

PART III

Sport-Specific Power Development

CHAPTER 9

Team Sport Power Training

Mike R. McGuigan,
PhD, CSCS

This chapter presents and discusses sample power training sessions and training programs for specific team sports. These sample sessions highlight the link between assessment and training. Coaches and athletes can use the samples here to help guide the development of training programs and individual training sessions. The reader should also review the practical case studies and examples presented in chapter 2 (methods of power assessment), chapter 3 (overall program periodization and integration of power), and chapter 4 (training programs for youth athletes and older populations).

These sample programs are presented in the context of training power and, for the most part, do not include extensive details on other aspects of the training plan. When putting together an overall training program, it is critical that practitioners take into account the other aspects of training that will affect the development and optimization of muscular power. The aspects of long-term planning discussed in chapter 3 need to be considered when designing power assessment and training programming.

Understanding the specific needs of the sport with which you are involved is necessary for designing position-specific training programs for power development. An important factor in training for team sports is the substantial differences in power needs between positions within a sport. For example, in a sport like rugby union, clear differences exist in the demands of a winger compared to those of a front-row forward. In American football, a lineman has different physical requirements than a wide receiver. A goalkeeper in soccer requires a different training approach than a midfield player. Prescribing training programs and exercises based on the demands of a position prepares the athlete for the specific demands of his or her role in competition and facilitates optimal performance. Along with selecting appropriate tests of physical capacity (chapter 2), the needs analysis should also include performance analysis of athletes during competition. This allows the coach to develop individualized training programs to meet the specific demands of the sport.

Another consideration when developing a training program for team sports is the complexity of the competitive season. Numerous competitions and long seasons can make designing a training program difficult. Additional factors must be considered: training age, game exposure, strengths and weaknesses (determined from fitness testing), injury history, and alterations in recent training load. All of these factors should influence the specific, individual plan for a player from a training (e.g., content and load) and game exposure perspective.

When using the templates and examples, it is critical to include an adequate warm-up for each training session. Examples of warm-ups for training sessions are provided in chapter 4.

RUGBY UNION

Power is a critical component of performance for collision-based team sports such as rugby. One approach to maximizing strength and power is to use a program template that emphasizes strength development one day and power development another. However, be sure to use the templates to develop programs that are relevant to the sport and athlete. Table 9.1 shows a 6-week training program for an intermediate-level rugby union player using a linear progression across the weeks. Exercises can be rotated in and out of the program using an appropriate combination of sets, repetitions, and percent of maximum. For example, on day 1, the back squat could be replaced with the front squat. For practitioners working with athletes who regularly compete once a week during the competition phase, high-force contrast training consisting of a heavy day and lighter day is an effective method for improving performance over a short training phase during the competitive season (1).

Power priming is used the day of or the day before a match to bring about a substantial improvement in performance (3). These sessions, designed with the needs of the athlete and sport in mind, are typically performed 5-24 hours before a match and last just 10-30 min. Table 9.2 shows a sample power priming session that emphasizes force and velocity for a rugby union athlete 6 hours before the match. In this session, the first two exercises are performed as a complex (sets of heavy resistance loads followed by sets of plyometric exercise). Other examples of strength–power potentiating complexes are shown in table 3.3 and further examples of exercise pairings are given in table 8.1.

BASKETBALL

The strength and conditioning practitioner is faced with significant challenges when programming for team sports. Sports such as basketball require a range of

Table 9.1 2-Day per Week, 6-Week Training Program for Intermediate-Level Rugby Union Player

DAY 1: STRENGTH						
Exercise	Week 1	Week 2	Week 3	Week 4	Week 5	Week 6
Bench press	3 × 6 (65%)	3 × 6 (75%)	3 × 6 (80%)	3 × 5 (85%)	3 × 3 (87.5%)	3 × 3 (90%)
Bench row	3 × 6 (65%)	3 × 6 (75%)	3 × 6 (80%)	3 × 5 (85%)	3 × 3 (87.5%)	3 × 3 (90%)
Back squat	3 × 6 (65%)	3 × 6 (75%)	3 × 6 (80%)	3 × 5 (85%)	3 × 3 (87.5%)	3 × 3 (90%)
Barbell push press	3 × 5 (65%)	3 × 5 (75%)	3 × 5 (77.5%)	3 × 5 (80%)	3 × 5 (85%)	3 × 5 (87.5%)
DAY 2: POWER						
Exercise	Week 1	Week 2	Week 3	Week 4	Week 5	Week 6
Jump squat	3 × 5 (30%)	3 × 5 (35%)	3 × 3 (40%)	3 × 5 (BW)	6 × 3 (BW)	10 × 2 (BW)
Front squat	3 × 6 (70%)	3 × 5 (75%)	3 × 5 (80%)	3 × 3 (82.5%)	3 × 3 (87.5%)	3 × 3 (90%)
Bench press throw	3 × 6 (30%)	3 × 5 (32.5%)	3 × 5 (35%)	3 × 3 (37.5%)	3 × 3 (40%)	3 × 2 (42.5%)
Barbell power jerk	3 × 6 (65%)	3 × 5 (70%)	3 × 5 (75%)	3 × 3 (80%)	3 × 3 (82.5%)	3 × 3 (85%)

BW = body weight; % refers to %1RM

Table 9.2 Sample Power Priming Workout for Rugby Union

Exercise	Sets × reps	Intensity
Back squat	3 × 3	85% 1RM
Jump squat*	3 × 3	BW
Band push-up	3 × 5	Max speed

*Back squat and jump squat could be performed as a contrast training complex with 2 min rest between alternating sets of each exercise.

BW = body weight

physical capacities in addition to power. Table 9.3 outlines a sample power training session for basketball players of all positions. A relatively small number of exercises are prescribed and repetitions are kept low to enable to the athlete to maximize power and velocity over the set. Practitioners could also incorporate an exercise that uses higher loads (≥85% 1RM) to improve strength. This is a good example of a mixed-methods training approach (chapter 3) and it has been shown to be an effective strategy for improving power in athletes (4).

Figure 9.1 shows a power profile for a basketball player. Based on the results of the testing, the athlete has good strength levels (as indicated by the 1RM squat and

Table 9.3 Sample Power Workout for Basketball Players

Exercise	Sets × reps	Intensity
Jump squat	3 × 5	20% 1RM
Power clean from hang	5 × 3	85% 1RM
Bench press	4 × 3	50% 1RM
Barbell push press	3 × 5	70% 1RM

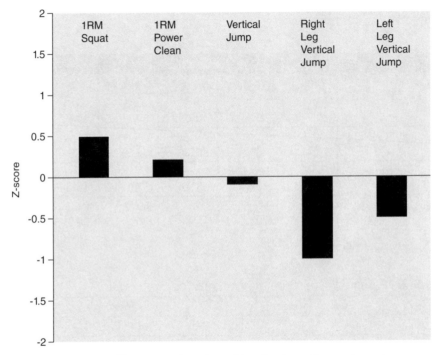

Figure 9.1 Power profile comparing the athlete's strengths and weaknesses using standardized Z-scores.

power clean results) but below-average vertical jump power (measured by jump height), particularly when tested on each leg. This testing shows the practitioner the specific areas that need attention, and the practitioner may decide to implement more single-leg training and also increase the amount of right-leg work to overcome the imbalance revealed by the testing.

SOCCER

Competitive seasons for many sports are becoming increasingly longer. This presents challenges for strength and conditioning practitioners both in terms of programming for power and how to maintain it throughout the competitive season. As discussed extensively in chapters 1 and 3, it is critical to maintain strength because it is the foundation of power. Resistance training should be a

Table 9.4 In-Season Power Training Program for a Soccer Player

DAY 1: POWER								
Exercise	Week 1	Week 2	Week 3	Week 4	Week 5	Week 6	Week 7	Week 8
Jump squat	3 × 5 (25%)	3 × 5 (30%-35%)	3 × 3 (35%-40%)	4 × 3 (BW)	3 × 5 (25%-30%)	5 × 3 (30%-35%)	6 × 2 (35%-40%)	6 × 2 (BW)
Back squat	3 × 6 (65%)	3 × 6 (70%)	3 × 5 (75%)	3 × 3 (80%)	3 × 6 (70%)	3 × 5 (75%)	3 × 3 (80%)	3 × 2 (85%)
Fast clean pull	4 × 5 (60%)	4 × 5 (65%)	4 × 5 (70%)		3 × 3 (70%)	3 × 3 (75%)	3 × 2 (80%)	
Dumbbell power clean to jerk	3 × 5 (20 kg [44 lb])	3 × 3 (30 kg [66 lb])	3 × 3 (35 kg [77 lb])	3 × 2 (40 kg [88 lb])	3 × 5 (25 kg [55 lb])	3 × 3 (30 kg [66 lb])	3 × 3 (35 kg [77 lb])	3 × 2 (30, 35, 40 kg [66, 77, 88 lb])
DAY 2: STRENGTH								
Exercise	Week 1	Week 2	Week 3	Week 4	Week 5	Week 6	Week 7	Week 8
Front squat	3 × 6 (70%)	3 × 6 (70%-80%)	3 × 5 (80%-85%)	3 × 3-5 (85%-90%)	3 × 6 (72.5%)	3 × 6 (70%-80%)	3 × 5 (80%-87.5%)	3 × 2-3 (90%-92.5%)
Squat jump*	3 × 3 (BW)	3 × 3 (BW)	3 × 3 (BW)		3 × 3 (BW)	3 × 3 (BW)	3 × 3 (BW)	3 × 3 (BW)
Bench press	3 × 6 (70%)	3 × 6 (70-80%)	3 × 5 (80-85%)	3 × 3-5 (85-90%)	3 × 6 (72.5%)	3 × 6 (70-80%)	3 × 5 (80-87.5%)	3 × 2-3 (90-92.5%)
Wood chop	3 × 5 (5 kg [11 lb])	3 × 3 (7 kg [15 lb])	3 × 2 (10 kg [22 lb])		3 × 5 (5 kg [11 lb])	3 × 3 (7 kg [15 lb])	3 × 2 (10 kg [22 lb])	

*Performed as a complex with front squat. BW = body weight; % refers to %1RM.

regular fixture for team sports because of the strong relationships between power and sprint and jump performance (chapters 1 and 2). Table 9.4 shows an example of an in-season power training program for an elite soccer player with the goal of maintaining power. This program uses a wavelike approach, including a week with decreased volume to provide variety (chapter 3).

AMERICAN FOOTBALL

This case study of a skill position player discusses an original program and adjustments based on a power profile (figure 9.2). The athlete is a wide receiver (age = 19 years, height = 1.85 m [6 ft], weight = 81.6 kg [180 lb]) and his coaches are concerned that he seems to have lost his ability to beat the opposition defender in a one-on-one situation. His speed and his ability to change direction have declined from earlier in the season. His power profile toward the end of training camp in August indicates that his strength levels are good (1RM squat = 190 kg [419 lb]),

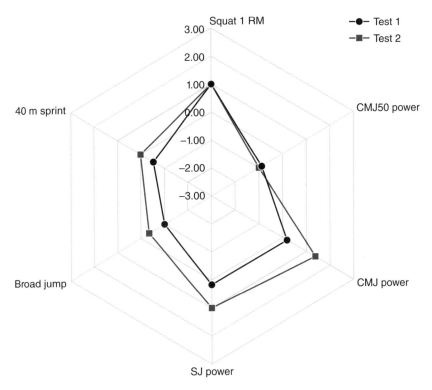

Figure 9.2 Power profile comparing the athlete's strengths and weaknesses using standardized Z-scores. CMJ = countermovement jump; SJ = static jump; CMJ50 = loaded countermovement jump (50 kg [110 lb]).

but his power capabilities during the 50 kg [110 lb] squat jump (40.5 W/kg) are poor. In addition, his vertical countermovement jump (CMJ) power (63 W/kg), reactive strength of 1.75 determined from drop jump test), and sprint ability (40 m time = 2.75 s) are below what was expected. In the 4 weeks before the August testing, the athlete performed three resistance training sessions per week. These sessions included a session of heavy clean pulls, squats (4 sets of 3 repetitions), Nordic hamstring drops (3 sets of 8 repetitions), lunges (3 sets of 10 repetitions), and upper body work performed early each week on Mondays. This was followed by a power day, consisting of hang snatches, 60 kg (132 lb) jump squats, and power cleans (4 sets of 3 repetitions), performed on Thursdays, and a whole-body hypertrophy session toward the end of the week.

Based on the information from the coaches and the results of the fitness testing, an adjustment to the weekly training program was made. For the first session each week, the athlete performed strength–power potentiation complexes including heavy back squats with depth jumps (50 cm [20 in]) and heavy clean pulls with repeated broad jumps (continuous, 3 sets of 4 repetitions followed with 3-5 jumps), upper body work (bench press, bench pull), and accessory exercises (abdominals). In the second session, the athlete completed the same power-based session, with the addition of box jumps, assisted jumps, and resisted jumps (3 sets of 3 repetitions) followed by agility ladder work and change-in-direction tasks (10 repetitions). The athlete performed this training program for three months. The athlete increased body-weight CMJ power (70 W/kg) and sprint ability (40 m time = 2.45 s), while maintaining maximum strength and loaded-CMJ power. It appears that the modifications in the training program improved his power capabilities. The hypertrophy session was removed to allow for greater focus on strength and power exercises. Specifically, the addition of strength–power potentiation complexes enabled lower body power to increase. Along with the addition of jumping and agility exercises, this transferred into speed improvements.

VOLLEYBALL

In sports such as volleyball, athletes complete a large volume of power-type movements, such as jumping, in training and competition. Therefore, practitioners need to be aware of this when designing power training programs for these sports. Large quantities of plyometric movements are not necessary in training sessions when athletes perform hundreds of these movements in training sessions. Loaded jumping through squat jumps using additional loads can be an effective way for athletes to improve jump performance (chapter 6). In this example, an elite volleyball player weighing 75 kg (165 lb) underwent a 6-week training program to increase her jump performance. Table 9.5 provides a sample progression in which moderate

Table 9.5 Six-Week Lower Body Strength and Power Training Program for an Elite Volleyball Player

SESSION 1						
Exercise	Week 1	Week 2	Week 3	Week 4	Week 5	Week 6
Jump squat	4 × 5 (20 kg [44 lb])	4 × 3 (30 kg [66 lb])	4 × 2 (40 kg [88 lb])	5 × 3 (20 kg [44 lb])	6 × 3 (15 kg [33 lb])	6 × 2 (10 kg [22 lb])
Power clean	5 × 3 (40 kg [88 lb])	6 × 3 (45 kg [99 lb])	6 × 2 (50 kg [110 lb])	5 × 2 (45 kg [99 lb])	6 × 3 (55 kg [121 lb])	6 × 2 (60 kg [132 lb])
Front squat	4 × 5 (45 kg [99 lb])	5 × 5 (50 kg [110 lb])	5 × 3 (55 kg [121 lb])		5 × 3 (55 kg [121 lb])	5 × 2 (60 kg [132 lb])
SESSION 2						
Exercise	Week 1	Week 2	Week 3	Week 4	Week 5	Week 6
Jump squat	4 × 4 (25 kg [55 lb])	5 × 3 (35 kg [77 lb])	6 × 2 (45 kg [99 lb])	6 × 3 (0 kg)	5 × 3 (0 kg)	6 × 2 (0 kg)
Power snatch	5 × 3 (30 kg [66 lb])	6 × 3 (35 kg [77 lb])	6 × 2 (40 kg [88 lb])	5 × 2 (35 kg [77 lb])	6 × 3 (40 kg [88 lb])	6 × 2 (45 kg [99 lb])
Back squat	5 × 3 (55 kg [121 lb])	6 × 3 (65 kg [143 lb])	6 × 2 (70 kg [154 lb])		6 × 3 (70 kg [154 lb])	6 × 3 (80 kg [176 lb])

(25%-75% of the athlete's mass) barbell loads in the jump squat are used initially and then reduced to relatively light-load jump squats (<25% of the athlete's mass). This loading progression in the jump squat can result in excellent improvements in jumping performance. The testing for this athlete could also include an investigation of impulse (force × time) or the way the athlete jumps if that technology, for example, a force plate or a contact mat, is available (figure 2.5).

BASEBALL

Baseball is another sport in which the physical demands are unique depending on the position and the role of the player. Practitioners should design training programs and sessions to develop power with this in mind. Table 9.6 outlines a power training session for a pitcher. Alternative approaches could be the use of ascending and descending power workouts as shown in tables 3.4 and 3.5. The practitioner should take into account the total number of throws the pitcher performs during all training sessions and games when designing these programs (2).

Table 9.6   Upper Body Power Training Session for a Baseball Player

Exercise	Sets × reps	Intensity
Band push-up	4 × 3-5	Increase loading via bands across the sets
Band row	3 × 6	Increase loading via bands across the sets
Lateral toss	3 × 6	3, 4, 5 kg (6.6, 8.8, 11 lb)
Single-arm dumbbell snatch	4 × 5	15, 20, 25, 30 kg (33, 44, 55, 66 lb)
Ball drop	4 × 3	3, 5, 7 kg (6.6, 11, 15 lb)

CONCLUSION

Practitioners are faced with unique challenges when designing training programs for team sports. Factors such as position demands, structure of the competitive season, training age, game exposure, strengths and weaknesses (determined from fitness testing), injury history, and alterations in recent training load need to be considered. Most critical is appreciating how power training fits within the overall physical preparation of the athlete and how assessment of power can be used to inform the training program design.

CHAPTER 10

Individual Sport Power Training

Mike R. McGuigan,
PhD, CSCS

This chapter provides examples of power training programs for a variety of individual sports, including track and field, swimming, wrestling, golf, rowing, and winter sports. As with the previous chapter, these programs highlight the link between assessment of power and how that assessment can be used to develop training programs.

The principles discussed at the beginning of chapter 9 also apply when dealing with individual sports. The strength and conditioning practitioner needs to be aware of the wide range of disciplines and events within these sports and take into account the specific needs of the athletes and their event, discipline, and sport when putting together both an individual session and a training program to improve power. The practitioner also needs to consider how the power training component fits within the overall training plan and conduct a thorough needs analysis of the sport and event to determine what physical qualities need to be trained. Maintenance of power during the competitive season should also be considered.

TRACK AND FIELD

This case study discusses a junior-level shot putter (age = 18 years, height = 1.8 m [5 ft 9 in], weight = 85 kg [187 lb]). The technical coach and the strength and conditioning practitioner have identified that the athlete needs to improve her explosiveness because they believe this will help increase her throwing distance. The athlete's power profile during November testing indicates that she is very strong (back squat 1RM = 130 kg [287 lb]) with average to below average explosive capabilities during the 40 kg (88 lb) squat jump (relative peak power = 24 W/kg), body-weight squat jump (relative peak power = 35 W/kg) and drop jump (reactive strength = 1.5). During the 4 weeks before the November testing, the athlete had been performing one heavy strength session that included back squats, deadlifts, and snatch pulls from blocks (6, 5, 3, 3 repetitions for the 4 weeks) on Mondays week, followed by a power day consisting of the full snatches, front squats, and power cleans (4 sets of 3 repetitions) later in the week (e.g., Thursday), in addition to a moderately heavy strength session that included upper body exercises.

Based on the results of the testing, the coaches adjusted her lower body lifting program. Her first session each week consisted of heavy back squats, snatch pulls, and push press (5 sets of 3 repetitions). The second session continued the same power session as before, but with the addition of a 30-50 kg (66-110 lb) loaded countermovement jump (4 sets of 3 repetitions). She performed this training program for 3 months. The results of the follow-up testing are outlined in figure 10.1. The athlete continued to increased her strength (1RM squat = 140 kg [309 lb]) and power capabilities during the 40 kg (88 lb) squat jump (30 W/kg) and maintained body-weight squat, countermovement, and drop jump (reactive strength) performance. Most important, her throwing distances in training improved by an average of 2%-3%. It appears that the modifications to the training program improved her strength and loaded-power capabilities while maintaining light-load velocity and power capabilities, which translated into increased sport performance. Focusing on how physical training can improve sport performance is the key for strength and conditioning practitioners.

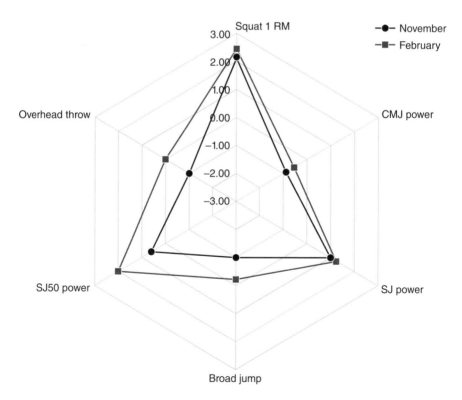

Figure 10.1 Power profile comparing the athlete's strengths and weaknesses using standardized Z-scores SJ50 power = loaded static jump (50 kg [110 lb]).

Table 10.1 outlines a power training program for a heptathlete. Multievents present significant challenges to coaches, who must manage the technical skill demands of the different events when scheduling the various disciplines during training sessions. In this sample program, the power-focused sessions are scheduled early in the week while the athlete is relatively fresh. The second session later in the week also focuses on power and also works on strength. The single-leg broad jump was added to the program after testing showed that distance on the single-leg horizontal jump test was lower than expected.

Table 10.1 Eight-Week Preseason Power Training Program for a Heptathlete

DAY 1: POWER								
Exercise	Week 1	Week 2	Week 3	Week 4	Week 5	Week 6	Week 7	Week 8
Squat jump	3 × 5 (25%)	3 × 5 (30%-35%)	3 × 3 (35%-40%)	4 × 3 (0%)	3 × 5 (25%-30%)	5 × 3 (30%-35%)	6 × 2 (35%-40%)	6 × 2 (0%)
Back squat	3 × 6 (65%)	3 × 6 (70%)	3 × 5 (75%)	3 × 3 (80%)	3 × 6 (70%)	3 × 5 (75%)	3 × 3 (80%)	3 × 2 (85%)
Fast snatch pull from blocks	4 × 5 (60%)	4 × 5 (65%)	4 × 5 (70%)		3 × 3 (70%)	3 × 3 (75%)	3 × 2 (80%)	
Dumbbell power clean to jerk	3 × 5 (20 kg [44lb])	3 × 3 (30 kg [66 lb])	3 × 3 (35 kg [77 lb])	3 × 2 (40 kg [88 lb])	3 × 5 (25 kg [55 lb])	3 × 3 (30 kg [66 lb])	3 × 3 (35 kg [77 lb])	3 × 2 (35,40, 45 kg [77, 88, 99 lb])
Overhead throw*	3 × 5 (4 kg [8.8 lb])	3 × 3 (5 kg [11 lb])	3 × 3 (6 kg [13 lb])	3 × 2 (4 kg [8.8 lb])	3 × 5 (4 kg [8.8 lb])	3 × 3 (3 kg [6.6 lb])	3 × 3 (5 kg [11 lb])	3 × 2 (4 kg [8.8 lb])
DAY 2: STRENGTH AND POWER								
Exercise	Week 1	Week 2	Week 3	Week 4	Week 5	Week 6	Week 7	Week 8
Front squat	3 × 6 (70%)	3 × 6 (70%-80%)	3 × 5 (80%-85%)	3 × 3-5 (85%-90%)	3 × 6 (72.5%)	3 × 6 (70%-80%)	3 × 5 (80%-87.5%)	3 × 2-3 (90%-92.5%)
Jump squat**	3 × 3 (BW)	3 × 3 (BW)	3 × 3 (BW)		3 × 3 (BW)	3 × 3 (BW)	3 × 3 (BW)	3 × 3 (BW)
Band bench press	3 × 6 (70%)	3 × 6 (70%-80%)	3 × 5 (80%-85%)	3 × 3-5 (85%-90%)	3 × 6 (72.5%)	3 × 6 (70%-80%)	3 × 5 (80%-87.5%)	3 × 2-3 (90%-92.5%)
Ball drop	3 × 5 (5 kg [11 lb])	3 × 3 (7 kg [15 lb])	3 × 2 (10 kg [22 lb])		3 × 5 (5 kg [11 lb])	3 × 3 (7 kg [15 lb])	3 × 2 (10 kg [22 lb])	

*Performed as a complex with dumbbell power clean to jerk.

**Performed as a complex with front squat.

BW = body weight

% Refers to %1RM

SWIMMING

As discussed in chapter 9, a power primer session provides an acute neuromuscular and hormonal effect before competition (or an important training session). It also provides the strength and conditioning coach an opportunity to include an additional training stimulus that is brief and intense for less experienced athletes (4). Table 10.2 outlines a power priming session for a sprint swimmer 24 hours before a meet. This session was developed through a process of trial and error early in the periodized program; different types of sessions were tested before less important races and training sessions.

Table 10.2 Sample Power Priming Workout for a Sprint Swimmer

Exercise	Sets × reps	Intensity
Squat jump	4 × 3	BW
Depth jump	3 × 3	45cm (18 in) box
Assisted jump	3 × 3	Using bands
Assisted band push-up	4 × 3	Using bands

BW = body weight

WRESTLING

In many sports, the ability to produce power repeatedly is important (chapter 2). This has led to the belief that circuit training with a focus on high repetitions and short rest periods (metabolic conditioning) can improve power and maintain it over the course of an event. However, research to support this is lacking, and in most cases, this type of training is not relevant to the athlete or is not sport specific. Table 10.3 shows a circuit in which a wrestler rotates through various stations while maintaining power output and session quality. In a sport such as wrestling, the athlete should obtain more than adequate amounts of metabolic conditioning from the sport-specific training sessions.

Table 10.3 Sample Power Circuit for a Wrestler

Exercise	Sets × reps	Intensity or time
Jump squat	4 × 6	BW
Band push-up	4 × 6	Light band
Single-arm dumbbell snatch	4 × 5	20-30 kg (44-66 lb)
Scoop toss	4 × 5	4 kg (8.8 lb)
Squat jump	4 × 6	BW
Jump push-up	4 × 5	Fast as possible
Dumbbell power clean to power jerk	4 × 5	25-35 kg (55-77 lb)
Overhead throw	4 × 5	4 kg (8.8 lb)
Abdominal twist	4 × 6	3 kg (6.6 lb)

BW = body weight
Athlete takes at least 30 s rest between stations.

GOLF

Power is important in the sport of golf (6). The ability to store and release elastic energy is a critical component of an effective golf swing. Table 10.4 outlines a training session that could be used to improve a golfer's power. Other options for rotational and upper body exercises are given in chapter 5.

Table 10.4 Sample Training Session for a Golfer

Exercise	Sets × reps	Intensity or time
Jump squat	4 × 5	BW
Loaded jump squat	4 × 3	20%, 25%, 30% 1RM
Bench press throw	4 × 5	30%, 35%, 40% 1RM
Push press	3 × 3	50%, 55%, 60% 1RM
Wood chop	3 × 5	4 kg (8.8 lb)
Abdominal twist	3 × 6	3 kg (6.6 lb)

ROWING

It is now well established that endurance sports can benefit from resistance training (1, 2). The sport of rowing requires muscular strength, endurance, and power. For endurance sports such as rowing, high repetitions with low loads are of little value and will not improve power (5). Therefore, the power training principles discussed in previous chapters apply here. Table 10.5 shows a 6-week training program for an elite rower. Rowers can also use cluster sets. Figure 3.21 and table 3.2 show examples of configurations for cluster sets.

In the following case study, a rower is tested using a 1 RM bench press, bench pull, power clean, and peak velocity on a bench press and bench pull with 40 kg (88 lb). The results showed a difference between the pushing and pulling strength and below-average velocity for both. This indicates that the emphasis of subsequent training should be on incorporating more pulling movements, such as rows and pulls, as well as an increased focus on lighter loads that can be moved at greater velocity.

WINTER SPORTS

Among the large variety of winter sports, power is important for many of them (3, 7). Table 10.6 shows a training session for a skeleton competitor. The strength and conditioning coach used 3 RM back squat and vertical jump to assess the athlete's strength and power. The latest round of testing identified that maximum strength is above average for this athlete, but the jump height is below average, which indicates that power is an issue that needs to be addressed. One of the sessions that the strength and conditioning practitioner implemented was a complex session to

Table 10.5 Two Day per Week, Six-Week Training Program for a Rower

DAY 1: STRENGTH						
Exercise	Week 1	Week 2	Week 3	Week 4	Week 5	Week 6
Bench press	3 × 6 (65%)	3 × 6 (75%)	3 × 6 (80%)	3 × 5 (85%)	3 × 3 (87.5%)	3 × 3 (90%)
Bench row	3 × 6 (70%)	3 × 6 (75%)	3 × 6 (80%)	3 × 5 (85%)	3 × 3 (87.5%)	3 × 3 (90%)
Back squat	3 × 6 (70%)	3 × 6 (75%)	3 × 6 (80%)	3 × 5 (85%)	3 × 3 (87.5%)	3 × 3 (90%)
Barbell push press	3 × 6 (65%)	3 × 5 (70%)	3 × 5 (75%)	3 × 3 (80%)	3 × 3 (82.5%)	3 × 3 (85%)
DAY 2: POWER						
Exercise	Week 1	Week 2	Week 3	Week 4	Week 5	Week 6
Squat jump	3 × 5 (30%)	3 × 5 (35%)	3 × 3 (40%)	3 × 5 (BW)	6 × 3 (BW)	8 × 2 (BW)
Front squat	3 × 6 (55%)	3 × 6 (60%)	3 × 6 (62.5%)	3 × 5 (65%)	3 × 4 (70%)	3 × 3 (75%)
Bench throw	3 × 5 (30%)	3 × 5 (32.5%)	3 × 5 (35%)	3 × 3 (37.5%)	3 × 3 (40%)	3 × 2 (42.5%)
Jump push-up	3 × 3	3 × 4	3 × 5	4 × 4	4 × 5	5 × 5

BW = body weight

Table 10.6 Sample Power Training Session for a Skeleton Athlete

Exercise	Sets × reps	Intensity
Back squat	4 × 3	90% 1RM
Squat jump*	4 × 3	BW
Heavy snatch pull from floor	3 × 3	85% 1RM
Broad jump**	3 × 3	BW
Barbell power jerk	3 × 5	80%-90% 1RM
Depth jump	3 × 3	40, 45, 50 cm (16, 18, 20 in) box

*Performed as a complex with back squat (3 min rest between exercises).
**Performed as a complex with heavy snatch pull (3 min rest between exercises).
BW = body weight

maintain strength but also increase power. The practitioner could also consider using strength–power potentiation complexes within in these types of sessions. Examples of these are shown in table 3.3.

MONITORING POWER TRAINING

Monitoring power and other variables during training sessions using technology such as linear position transducers, force plates, and accelerometers is becoming increasingly common in sport settings. As discussed in chapter 8, methods such as velocity-based training are becoming more widely used, and they provide innovative ways to determine optimal resistance training loads through feedback. For the practitioner who has access to technology that can accurately measure velocity, figure 8.7 provides a general guideline for establishing training zones from testing data.

Practitioners may also use the information obtained from these technologies as an indicator of neuromuscular fatigue and the athlete's readiness to train. However, only a small body of research makes evidence-based recommendations for accurately using this type of information in practice (see chapter 8). The following is an example of how to use this approach for a downhill skier. Before the start of each power training session, the athlete performs a series of three squat jumps. A transducer measures mean power output for the jumps. Power testing performed early in the training cycle determined a baseline (2,000 W) and power testing established the smallest worthwhile change (140 W). Therefore, if monitoring produces a result below this threshold (1,860 W), it could be an indication of fatigue. The practitioner considers this information in the context of other monitoring information obtained, such as results of a wellness questionnaire or asking the athlete how he or she feels. The practitioner now has a decision to make: continue with the power training session as planned or modify the session. For example, the practitioner may decide to reduce the number of exercises, sets, or repetitions in order to maintain the quality of the session. This could involve monitoring the power of each repetition if the technology is available. This type of objective information from power monitoring can provide the practitioner with additional insights into the programming and allow the practitioner to adjust the session as it progresses. The challenge for practitioners is using this information without losing sight of the primary goal: using the information to improve the performance of the athlete or client.

CONCLUSION

Practitioners can use a range of tests to assess power in their athletes. Many training techniques are available to improve power. The link between testing and programming, that is, how the results of the testing influence the training program design, is critical. It is also important to remember that power development is just one piece of the training puzzle, and it needs to be put in the context of the overall training prescription. Understanding the assessments, training methods, and periodization specific to the needs of the athlete and the sport will help practitioners optimize their training programs.

References

Chapter 1

1. Aagaard P, Andersen JL, Dyhre-Poulsen P, Leffers AM, Wagner A, Magnusson SP, Halkjaer-Kristensen J, and Simonsen EB. A mechanism for increased contractile strength of human pennate muscle in response to strength training: changes in muscle architecture. *J Physiol* 534: 613-623, 2001.

2. Ackland DC, Lin YC, and Pandy MG. Sensitivity of model predictions of muscle function to changes in moment arms and muscle-tendon properties: a Monte-Carlo analysis. *J Biomech* 45: 1463-1471, 2012.

3. Arnold EM, Hamner SR, Seth A, Millard M, and Delp SL. How muscle fiber lengths and velocities affect muscle force generation as humans walk and run at different speeds. *J Exp Biol* 216: 2150-2160, 2013.

4. Askew GN and Marsh RL. Optimal shortening velocity (V/Vmax) of skeletal muscle during cyclical contractions: length-force effects and velocity-dependent activation and deactivation. *J Exp Biol* 201: 1527-1540, 1998.

5. Avogadro P, Chaux C, Bourdin M, Dalleau G, and Belli A. The use of treadmill ergometers for extensive calculation of external work and leg stiffness during running. *Eur J Appl Physiol* 92: 182-185, 2004.

6. Azizi E, Brainerd EL, and Roberts TJ. Variable gearing in pennate muscles. *Proc Natl Acad Sci U S A* 105: 1745-1750, 2008.

7. Barclay CJ, Woledge RC, and Curtin NA. Inferring crossbridge properties from skeletal muscle energetics. *Prog Biophys Mol Biol* 102: 53-71, 2010.

8. Baxter JR and Piazza SJ. Plantar flexor moment arm and muscle volume predict torque-generating capacity in young men. *J Appl Physiol* 116: 538-544, 2014.

9. Belli A, Kyrolainen H, and Komi PV. Moment and power of lower limb joints in running. *Int J Sports Med* 23: 136-141, 2002.

10. Biewener AA. Locomotion as an emergent property of muscle contractile dynamics. *J Exp Biol* 219: 285-294, 2016.

11. Bloemink MJ, Melkani GC, Bernstein SI, and Geeves MA. The relay/converter interface influences hydrolysis of ATP by skeletal muscle myosin II. *J Biol Chem* 291: 1763-1773, 2016.

12. Bottinelli R, Pellegrino MA, Canepari M, Rossi R, and Reggiani C. Specific contributions of various muscle fibre types to human muscle performance: an in vitro study. *J Electromyogr Kinesiol* 9: 87-95, 1999.

13. Brainerd EL and Azizi E. Muscle fiber angle, segment bulging and architectural gear ratio in segmented musculature. *J Exp Biol* 208: 3249-3261, 2005.

14. Burghardt TP, Hu JY, and Ajtai K. Myosin dynamics on the millisecond time scale. *Biophys Chem* 131: 15-28, 2007.

15. Cannon DT, Bimson WE, Hampson SA, Bowen TS, Murgatroyd SR, Marwood S, Kemp GJ, and Rossiter HB. Skeletal muscle ATP turnover by 31P magnetic resonance spectroscopy during moderate and heavy bilateral knee extension. *J Physiol* 592: 5287-5300, 2014.

16. Cavagna GA, Legramandi MA, and La Torre A. Running backwards: soft landing-hard takeoff, a less efficient rebound. *Proc Biol Sci* 278: 339-346, 2011.

17. Cavagna GA, Legramandi MA, and Peyre-Tartaruga LA. Old men running: mechanical work and elastic bounce. *Proc Biol Sci* 275: 411-418, 2008.

18. Cavagna GA, Zamboni A, Faraggiana T, and Margaria R. Jumping on the moon: power output at different gravity values. *Aerosp Med* 43: 408-414, 1972.

19. Coggan AR. Use of stable isotopes to study carbohydrate and fat metabolism at the whole-body level. *Proc Nutr Soc* 58: 953-961, 1999.

20. Cormie P, McBride JM, and McCaulley GO. Power-time, force-time, and velocity-time curve analysis during the jump squat: impact of load. *J Appl Biomech* 24: 112-120, 2008.

21. Cormie P, McCaulley GO, and McBride JM. Power versus strength-power jump squat training: influence on the load-power relationship. *Med Sci Sports Exerc* 39: 996-1003, 2007.

22. Cormie P, McCaulley GO, Triplett NT, and McBride JM. Optimal loading for maximal power output during lower-body resistance exercises. *Med Sci Sports Exerc* 39: 340-349, 2007.

23. Cornachione AS, Leite F, Bagni MA, and Rassier DE. The increase in non-cross-bridge forces after stretch of activated striated muscle is related to titin isoforms. *Am J Physiol Cell Physiol* 310:C19-26, 2016.

24. Croce R, Miller J, Chamberlin K, Filipovic D, and Smith W. Wavelet analysis of quadriceps power spectra and amplitude under varying levels of contraction intensity and velocity. *Muscle Nerve* 50: 844-853, 2014.

25. Davies CT and Young K. Effects of external loading on short term power output in children and young male adults. *Eur J Appl Physiol Occup Physiol* 52: 351-354, 1984.

26. Deschenes MR, Judelson DA, Kraemer WJ, Meskaitis VJ, Volek JS, Nindl BC, Harman FS, and Deaver DR. Effects of resistance training on neuromuscular junction morphology. *Muscle Nerve* 23: 1576-1581, 2000.

27. Desmedt JE and Godaux E. Ballistic contractions in man: characteristic recruitment pattern of single motor units of the tibialis anterior muscle. *J Physiol* 264: 673-693, 1977.

28. di Prampero PE and Ferretti G. The energetics of anaerobic muscle metabolism: a reappraisal of older and recent concepts. *Respir Physiol* 118: 103-115, 1999.

29. Diederichs F. From cycling between coupled reactions to the cross-bridge cycle: mechanical power output as an integral part of energy metabolism. *Metabolites* 2: 667-700, 2012.

30. Domire ZJ and Challis JH. Maximum height and minimum time vertical jumping. *J Biomech* 48: 2865-2870, 2015.

31. Findley T, Chaudhry H, and Dhar S. Transmission of muscle force to fascia during exercise. *J Bodyw Mov Ther* 19: 119-123, 2015.

32. Finni T, Ikegawa S, Lepola V, and Komi PV. Comparison of force-velocity relationships of vastus lateralis muscle in isokinetic and in stretch-shortening cycle exercises. *Acta Physiol Scand* 177: 483-491, 2003.

33. Fischer G, Storniolo JL, and Eyre-Tartaruga LA. Effects of fatigue on running mechanics: spring-mass behavior in recreational runners after 60 seconds of countermovement jumps. *J Appl Biomech* 31: 445-451, 2015.

34. Fitts RH, McDonald KS, and Schluter JM. The determinants of skeletal muscle force and power: their adaptability with changes in activity pattern. *J Biomech* 24 Suppl 1: 111-122, 1991.

35. Fitts RH and Widrick JJ. Muscle mechanics: adaptations with exercise-training. *Exerc Sport Sci Rev* 24: 427-473, 1996.

36. Gastin PB. Energy system interaction and relative contribution during maximal exercise. *Sports Med* 31: 725-741, 2001.

37. Giroux C, Rabita G, Chollet D, and Guilhem G. Optimal balance between force and velocity differs among world-class athletes. *J Appl Biomech* 32: 59-68, 2016.

38. Glancy B, Barstow T, and Willis WT. Linear relation between time constant of oxygen uptake kinetics, total creatine, and mitochondrial content in vitro. *Am J Physiol Cell Physiol* 294: C79-87, 2008.

39. Grahammer J. A review of power output studies of Olympic and powerlifting: methodology, performance prediction, and evaluation tests. *J Strength Cond Res* 7: 76-89, 1993.

40. Hamner SR and Delp SL. Muscle contributions to fore-aft and vertical body mass center accelerations over a range of running speeds. *J Biomech* 46: 780-787, 2013.

41. Harridge SD, Bottinelli R, Canepari M, Pellegrino M, Reggiani C, Esbjornsson M, Balsom PD, and Saltin B. Sprint training, in vitro and in vivo muscle function, and myosin heavy chain expression. *J Appl Physiol* 84: 442-449, 1998.

42. Harridge SD, Bottinelli R, Canepari M, Pellegrino MA, Reggiani C, Esbjornsson M, and Saltin B. Whole-muscle and single-fibre contractile properties and myosin heavy chain isoforms in humans. *Pflugers Arch* 432: 913-920, 1996.

43. Hashizume S, Iwanuma S, Akagi R, Kanehisa H, Kawakami Y, and Yanai T. The contraction-induced increase in Achilles tendon moment arm: a three-dimensional study. *J Biomech* 47: 3226-3231, 2014.

44. Hawley JA and Leckey JJ. Carbohydrate dependence during prolonged, intense endurance exercise. *Sports Med* 45 Suppl 1: 5-12, 2015.

45. Heise GD, Smith JD, and Martin PE. Lower extremity mechanical work during stance phase of running partially explains interindividual variability of metabolic power. *Eur J Appl Physiol* 111: 1777-1785, 2011.

46. Herbert RD, Moseley AM, Butler JE, and Gandevia SC. Change in length of relaxed muscle fascicles and tendons with knee and ankle movement in humans. *J Physiol* 539: 637-645, 2002.

47. Hintzy F, Mourot L, Perrey S, and Tordi N. Effect of endurance training on different mechanical efficiency indices during submaximal cycling in subjects unaccustomed to cycling. *Can J Appl Physiol* 30: 520-528, 2005.

48. Hori N, Newton RU, Andrews WA, Kawamori N, McGuigan MR, and Nosaka K. Comparison of four different methods to measure power output during the hang power clean and the weighted jump squat. *J Strength Cond Res* 21: 314-320, 2007.

49. Hunter SK, Thompson MW, Ruell PA, Harmer AR, Thom JM, Gwinn TH, and Adams RD. Human skeletal sarcoplasmic reticulum Ca2+ uptake and muscle function with aging and strength training. *J Appl Physiol* 86: 1858-1865, 1999.

50. Jimenez-Reyes P, Samozino P, Cuadrado-Penafiel V, Conceicao F, Gonzalez-Badillo JJ, and Morin JB. Effect of countermovement on power-force-velocity profile. *Eur J Appl Physiol* 114: 2281-2288, 2014.

51. Karatzaferi C, Chinn MK, and Cooke R. The force exerted by a muscle cross-bridge depends directly on the strength of the actomyosin bond. *Biophys J* 87: 2532-2544, 2004.

52. Kipp K, Harris C, and Sabick MB. Correlations between internal and external power outputs during weightlifting exercise. *J Strength Cond Res* 27: 1025-1030, 2013.

53. Kitamura K, Tokunaga M, Iwane AH, and Yanagida T. A single myosin head moves along an actin filament with regular steps of 5.3 nanometres. *Nature* 397: 129-134, 1999.

54. Krylow AM and Sandercock TG. Dynamic force responses of muscle involving eccentric contraction. *J Biomech* 30: 27-33, 1997.

55. Kyrolainen H and Komi PV. Differences in mechanical efficiency between power- and endurance-trained athletes while jumping. *Eur J Appl Physiol Occup Physiol* 70: 36-44, 1995.

56. Kyrolainen H, Komi PV, and Belli A. Mechanical efficiency in athletes during running. *Scand J Med Sci Sports* 5: 200-208, 1995.

57. Loturco I, Kobal R, Maldonado T, Piazzi AF, Bottino A, Kitamura K, Abad CC, Pereira LA, and Nakamura FY. Jump squat is more related to sprinting and jumping abilities than Olympic push press. *Int J Sports Med* 2015. [e-pub ahead of print].

58. Loturco I, Nakamura FY, Artioli GG, Kobal R, Kitamura K, Cal Abad CC, Cruz IF, Romano F, Pereira LA, and Franchini E. Strength and power qualities are highly associated with punching impact in elite amateur boxers. *J Strength Cond Res* 30: 109-116, 2016.

59. Luhtanen P and Komi PV. Mechanical energy states during running. *Eur J Appl Physiol Occup Physiol* 38: 41-48, 1978.

60. Luhtanen P and Komi PV. Force-, power-, and elasticity-velocity relationships in walking, running, and jumping. *Eur J Appl Physiol Occup Physiol* 44: 279-289, 1980.

61. Mansson A, Rassier D, and Tsiavaliaris G. Poorly understood aspects of striated muscle contraction. *Biomed Res Int* 2015: 245154, 2015.

62. Markovic G and Jaric S. Positive and negative loading and mechanical output in maximum vertical jumping. *Med Sci Sports Exerc* 39: 1757-1764, 2007.

63. Martin PE, Heise GD, and Morgan DW. Interrelationships between mechanical power, energy transfers, and walking and running economy. *Med Sci Sports Exerc* 25: 508-515, 1993.

64. McBride JM, Haines TL, and Kirby TJ. Effect of loading on peak power of the bar, body, and system during power cleans, squats, and jump squats. *J Sports Sci* 29: 1215-1221, 2011.

65. McBride JM and Snyder JG. Mechanical efficiency and force-time curve variation during repetitive jumping in trained and untrained jumpers. *Eur J Appl Physiol* 112: 3469-3477, 2012.

66. Methenitis SK, Zaras ND, Spengos KM, Stasinaki AN, Karampatsos GP, Georgiadis GV, and Terzis GD. Role of muscle morphology in jumping, sprinting, and throwing performance in participants with different power training duration experience. *J Strength Cond Res* 30: 807-817, 2016.

67. Miller MS, Bedrin NG, Ades PA, Palmer BM, and Toth MJ. Molecular determinants of force production in human skeletal muscle fibers: effects of myosin isoform expression and cross-sectional area. *Am J Physiol Cell Physiol* 308: C473-484, 2015.

68. Miller MS, Bedrin NG, Callahan DM, Previs MJ, Jennings ME 2nd, Ades PA, Maughan DW, Palmer BM, and Toth MJ. Age-related slowing of myosin actin cross-bridge kinetics is sex specific and predicts decrements in whole skeletal muscle performance in humans. *J Appl Physiol* 115: 1004-1014, 2013.

69. Morel B, Rouffet DM, Saboul D, Rota S, Clemencon M, and Hautier CA. Peak torque and rate of torque development influence on repeated maximal exercise performance: contractile and neural contributions. *PloS one* 10:e0119719, 2015.

70. Nardello F, Ardigo LP, and Minetti AE. Measured and predicted mechanical internal work in human locomotion. *Hum Mov Sci* 30: 90-104, 2011.

71. Nuzzo JL, McBride JM, Dayne AM, Israetel MA, Dumke CL, and Triplett NT. Testing of the maximal dynamic output hypothesis in trained and untrained subjects. *J Strength Cond Res* 24: 1269-1276, 2010.

72. O'Brien TD, Reeves ND, Baltzopoulos V, Jones DA, and Maganaris CN. Strong relationships exist between muscle volume, joint power and whole-body external mechanical power in adults and children. *Exp Physiol* 94: 731-738, 2009.

73. Plas RL, Degens H, Meijer JP, de Wit GM, Philippens IH, Bobbert MF, and Jaspers RT. Muscle contractile properties as an explanation of the higher mean power output in marmosets than humans during jumping. *J Exp Biol* 218: 2166-2173, 2015.

74. Proske U and Allen TJ. Damage to skeletal muscle from eccentric exercise. *Exerc Sport Sci Rev* 33: 98-104, 2005.

75. Rassier DE, MacIntosh BR, and Herzog W. Length dependence of active force production in skeletal muscle. *J Appl Physiol* 86: 1445-1457, 1999.

76. Rubenson J, Lloyd DG, Heliams DB, Besier TF, and Fournier PA. Adaptations for economical bipedal running: the effect of limb structure on three-dimensional joint mechanics. *J R Soc Interface* 8: 740-755, 2011.

77. Sasaki K, Neptune RR, and Kautz SA. The relationships between muscle, external, internal and joint mechanical work during normal walking. *J Exp Biol* 212: 738-744, 2009.

78. Schache AG, Brown NA, and Pandy MG. Modulation of work and power by the human lower-limb joints with increasing steady-state locomotion speed. *J Exp Biol* 218: 2472-2481, 2015.

79. Scott CB. Contribution of blood lactate to the energy expenditure of weight training. *J Strength Cond Res* 20: 404-411, 2006.

80. Seebacher F, Tallis JA, and James RS. The cost of muscle power production: muscle oxygen consumption per unit work increases at low temperatures in Xenopus laevis. *J Exp Biol* 217: 1940-1945, 2014.

81. Shen ZH and Seipel JE. A fundamental mechanism of legged locomotion with hip torque and leg damping. *Bioinspir Biomim* 7:046010, 2012.

82. Smith DA. A new mechanokinetic model for muscle contraction, where force and movement are triggered by phosphate release. *J Muscle Res Cell Motil* 35: 295-306, 2014.

83. Snow DH, Harris RC, and Gash SP. Metabolic response of equine muscle to intermittent maximal exercise. *J Appl Physiol* 58: 1689-1697, 1985.

84. Sogaard K, Gandevia SC, Todd G, Petersen NT, and Taylor JL. The effect of sustained low-intensity contractions on supraspinal fatigue in human elbow flexor muscles. *J Physiol* 573: 511-523, 2006.

85. Soriano MA, Jimenez-Reyes P, Rhea MR, and Marin PJ. The optimal load for maximal power production during lower-body resistance exercises: a meta-analysis. *Sports Med* 45: 1191-1205, 2015.

86. Suzuki M, Fujita H, and Ishiwata S. A new muscle contractile system composed of a thick filament lattice and a single actin filament. *Biophys J* 89: 321-328, 2005.

87. Taboga P, Lazzer S, Fessehatsion R, Agosti F, Sartorio A, and di Prampero PE. Energetics and mechanics of running men: the influence of body mass. *Eur J Appl Physiol* 112: 4027-4033, 2012.

88. Toji H and Kaneko M. Effect of multiple-load training on the force-velocity relationship. *J Strength Cond Res* 18: 792-795, 2004.

89. Toji H, Suei K, and Kaneko M. Effects of combined training loads on relations among force, velocity, and power development. *Can J Appl Physiol* 22: 328-336, 1997.

90. Trappe S, Godard M, Gallagher P, Carroll C, Rowden G, and Porter D. Resistance training improves single muscle fiber contractile function in older women. *Am J Physiol Cell Physiol* 281: C398-406, 2001.

91. Van Cutsem M, Duchateau J, and Hainaut K. Changes in single motor unit behaviour contribute to the increase in contraction speed after dynamic training in humans. *J Physiol* 513 (Pt 1): 295-305, 1998.

92. Waterman-Storer CM. The cytoskeleton of skeletal muscle: is it affected by exercise? A brief review. *Med Sci Sports Exerc* 23: 1240-1249, 1991.

93. Willems PA, Cavagna GA, and Heglund NC. External, internal and total work in human locomotion. *J Exp Biol* 198: 379-393, 1995.

94. Williams PE and Goldspink G. Longitudinal growth of striated muscle fibres. *J Cell Sci* 9: 751-767, 1971.

95. Willis WT, Jackman MR, Messer JI, Kuzmiak-Glancy S, and Glancy B. A simple hydraulic analog model of oxidative phosphorylation. *Med Sci Sports Exerc 48: 990-1000, 2016.*

Chapter 2

1. Baker D and Newton RU. Methods to increase the effectiveness of maximal power training for the upper body. *Strength Cond J* 27: 24-32, 2005.

2. Bosco C, Luhtanen P, and Komi PV. A simple method for measurement of mechanical power in jumping. *Eur J Appl Physiol* 50: 273-282, 1983.

3. Chia M and Aziz AR. Modelling maximal oxygen uptake in athletes: allometric scaling versus ratio-scaling in relation to body mass. *Ann Acad Med Singapore* 37: 300-306, 2008.

4. Cormack SJ, Newton RU, McGuigan MR, and Doyle TLA. Reliability of measures obtained during single and repeated countermovement jumps. *Int J Sports Physiol Perform* 3: 131-144, 2008.

5. Cormie P, McBride JM, and McCaulley GO. Validation of power measurement technique in dynamic lower body resistance exercises. *J Appl Biomech* 23: 103-118, 2007.

6. Cormie P, McBride JM, and McCaulley GO. Power-time, force-time, and velocity-time curve analysis of the countermovement jump: impact of training. *J Strength Cond Res* 23: 177, 2009.

7. Cormie P, McCaulley GO, Triplett NT, and McBride JM. Optimal loading for maximal power output during lower-body resistance exercises. *Med Sci Sports Exerc* 39: 340-349, 2007.

8. Crewther BT, Kilduff LP, Cunningham DJ, Cook C, Owen N, and Yang GZ. Validating two systems for estimating force and power. *Int J Sports Med* 32: 254-258, 2011.

9. Crewther BT, McGuigan MR, and Gill ND. The ratio and allometric scaling of speed, power, and strength in elite male rugby union players. *J Strength Cond Res* 25: 1968-1975, 2011.

10. Cronin J and Sleivert G. Challenges in understanding the influence of maximal power training on improving athletic performance. *Sports Med* 35: 213-234, 2005.

11. Dugan EL, Doyle TL, Humphries B, Hasson CJ, and Newton RU. Determining the optimal load for jump squats: a review of methods and calculations. *J Strength Cond Res* 18: 668-674, 2004.

12. Fox, EL and Mathews, DK. *Interval Training: Conditioning for Sports and General Fitness.* Philadelphia, PA: Saunders, 1974. pp. 257-258.

13. Garhammer J. A review of power output studies of Olympic and powerlifting: methodology, performance prediction, and evaluation tests. *J Strength Cond Res* 7: 76-89, 1993.

14. Haff GG and Nimphius S. Training principles for power. *Strength Cond J* 34: 2-12, 2012.

15. Harman E, Rosenstein MT, Frykman PN, Rosenstein RM, and Kraemer WJ. Estimation of human power output from vertical jump. *J Appl Sport Sci Res* 5: 116-120, 1991.

16. Hopkins WG. How to interpret changes in an athletic performance test. *Sportscience* 8: 1-7, 2004.

17. Hopkins WG, Schabort EJ, and Hawley JA. Reliability of power in physical performance tests. *Sports Med* 31: 211-234, 2001.

18. Hori N, Newton RU, Andrews WA, Kawamori N, McGuigan MR, and Nosaka K. Comparison of four different methods to measure power output during the hang power clean and the weighted jump squat. *J Strength Cond Res* 21: 314-320, 2007.

19. Hori N, Newton RU, Kawamori N, McGuigan MR, Kraemer WJ, and Nosaka K. Reliability of performance measurements derived from ground reaction force data during countermovement jump and the influence of sampling frequency. *J Strength Cond Res* 23: 874-882, 2009.

20. Hori N, Newton RU, Nosaka K, and McGuigan MR. Comparison of different methods of determining power output in weightlifting exercises. *Strength Cond J* 28: 34-40, 2006.

21. Jaric S. Role of body size in the relation between muscle strength and movement performance. *Exerc Sport Sci Rev* 31: 8-12, 2003.

22. Knudson DV. Correcting the use of the term "power" in the strength and conditioning literature. *J Strength Cond Res* 23: 1902-1908, 2009.

23. McLellan CP, Lovell DI, and Gass GC. The role of rate of force development on vertical jump performance. *J Strength Cond Res* 25: 379-385, 2011.

24. McMaster DT, Gill N, Cronin J, and McGuigan M. A brief review of strength and ballistic assessment methodologies in sport. *Sports Med* 44: 603-623, 2014.

25. Moir GL, Gollie JM, Davis SE, Guers JJ, and Witmer CA. The effects of load on system and lower-body joint kinetics during jump squats. *Sports Biomech* 11: 492-506, 2012.

26. Nevill AM, Stewart AD, Olds T, and Holder R. Are adult physiques geometrically similar? The dangers of allometric scaling using body mass power laws. *Am J Phys Anthropol* 124: 177-182, 2004.

27. Nimphius S, McGuigan MR, and Newton RU. Relationship between strength, power, speed, and change of direction performance of female softball players. *J Strength Cond Res* 24: 885-895, 2010.

28. Nimphius S, McGuigan MR, and Newton RU. Changes in muscle architecture and performance during a competitive season in female softball players. *J Strength Cond Res* 26: 2655-2666, 2012.

29. Nuzzo JL, McBride JM, Cormie P, and McCaulley GO. Relationship between countermovement jump performance and multijoint isometric and dynamic tests of strength. *J Strength Cond Res* 22: 699-707, 2008.

30. Sayers SP, Harackiewicz DV, Harman EA, Frykman PN, and Rosenstein MT. Cross-validation of three jump power equations. *Med Sci Sports Exerc* 31: 572-577, 1999.

31. Stone MH, Stone M, and Sands WA. Testing, Measurement, and Evaluation, in: *Principles and Practices of Resistance Training*. Champaign, IL: Human Kinetics, 2007, pp 157-179.

32. Suchomel TJ, Nimphius S, and Stone MH. The importance of muscular strength in athletic performance. *Sports Med* 46: 1419-1449, 2016.

33. Tessier JF, Basset FA, Simoneau M, and Teasdale N. Lower-limb power cannot be estimated accurately from vertical jump tests. *J Hum Kinet* 38: 5-13, 2013.

34. Vanderburgh PM, Sharp M, and Nindl B. Nonparallel slopes using analysis of covariance for body size adjustment may reflect inappropriate modeling. *Meas Phys Educ Exerc Sci* 2: 127-135, 1998.

35. Wilson GJ, Newton RU, Murphy AJ, and Humphries BJ. The optimal training load for the development of dynamic athletic performance. *Med Sci Sports Exerc* 25: 1279-1286, 1993.

36. Winter EM, Abt G, Brookes FB, Challis JH, Fowler NE, Knudson DV, Knuttgen HG, Kraemer WJ, Lane AM, van Mechelen W, Morton RH, Newton RU, Williams C, and Yeadon MR. Misuse of "power" and other mechanical terms in sport and exercise science research. *J Strength Cond Res* 30: 292-300, 2016.

37. Zoeller RF, Ryan ED, Gordish-Dressman H, Price TB, Seip RL, Angelopoulos TJ, Moyna NM, Gordon PM, Thompson PD, and Hoffman EP. Allometric scaling of isometric biceps strength in adult females and the effect of body mass index. *Eur J Appl Physiol* 104: 701-710, 2008.

Chapter 3

1. Aagaard P, Simonsen EB, Andersen JL, Magnusson P, and Dyhre-Poulsen P. Increased rate of force development and neural drive of human skeletal muscle following resistance training. *J Appl Physiol* 93: 1318-1326, 2002.

2. Aagaard P, Simonsen EB, Andersen JL, Magnusson P, and Dyhre-Poulsen P. Neural adaptation to resistance training: changes in evoked V-wave and H-reflex responses. *J Appl Physiol* 92: 2309-2318, 2002.

3. Aagaard P, Simonsen EB, Trolle M, Bangsbo J, and Klausen K. Effects of different strength training regimes on moment and power generation during dynamic knee extensions. *Eur J Appl Physiol* 69: 382-386, 1994.

4. Baker D. Comparison of upper-body strength and power between professional and college-aged rugby league players. *J Strength Cond Res* 15: 30-35, 2001.

5. Baker D. A series of studies on the training of high-intensity muscle power in rugby league football players. *J Strength Cond Res* 15: 198-209, 2001.

6. Baker D, Wilson G, and Carlyon R. Periodization: the effect on strength of manipulating volume and intensity. *J Strength Cond Res* 8: 235-242, 1994.

7. Banister EW, Carter JB, and Zarkadas PC. Training theory and taper: validation in triathlon athletes. *Eur J Appl Physiol Occup Physiol* 79: 182-191, 1999.

8. Barker M, Wyatt TJ, Johnson RL, Stone MH, O'Bryant HS, Poe C, and Kent M. Performance factors, physiological assessment, physical characteristic, and football playing ability. *J Strength Cond Res* 7: 224-233, 1993.

9. Bartolomei S, Hoffman JR, Merni F, and Stout JR. A comparison of traditional and block periodized strength training programs in trained athletes. *J Strength Cond Res* 28: 990-997, 2014.

10. Bompa TO and Buzzichelli CA. Periodization as planning and programming of sport training, in: *Periodization Training for Sports*. Champaign, IL: Human Kinetics, 2015, pp 87-98.

11. Bompa TO and Haff GG. *Periodization: Theory and Methodology of Training*. Champaign, IL: Human Kinetics Publishers, 2009.

12. Bondarchuk A. *Transfer of Training in Sports*. Michigan, USA: Ultimate Athlete Concepts, 2007.

13. Bondarchuk AP. Track and field training. *Legkaya Atletika* 12: 8-9, 1986.

14. Bondarchuk AP. Constructing a Training System. *Track Tech* 102: 254-269, 1988.

15. Bondarchuk AP. The role and sequence of using different training-load intensities. *Fit Sports Rev Inter* 29: 202-204, 1994.

16. Bosquet L, Montpetit J, Arvisais D, and Mujika I. Effects of tapering on performance: a meta-analysis. *Med Sci Sports Exerc* 39: 1358-1365, 2007.

17. Bruin G, Kuipers H, Keizer HA, and Vander Vusse GJ. Adaptation and overtraining in horses subjected to increasing training loads. *J Appl Physiol* 76: 1908-1913, 1994.

18. Chiu LZF and Barnes JL. The fitness-fatigue model revistited: implications for planning short- and long-term training. *NSCA J* 25: 42-51, 2003.

19. Cormie P, McGuigan MR, and Newton RU. Adaptations in athletic performance following ballistic power vs strength training. *Med Sci Sports Exerc* 42: 1582-1598, 2010.

20. Cormie P, McGuigan MR, and Newton RU. Influence of strength on magnitude and mechanisms of adaptation to power training. *Med Sci Sports Exerc* 42: 1566-1581, 2010.

21. Cormie P, McGuigan MR, and Newton RU. Developing maximal neuromuscular power. Part II: training considerations for improving maximal power production. *Sports Med* 41: 125-146, 2011.

22. Counsilman JE and Counsilman BE. *The New Science of Swimming*. Englewood Cliffs, NJ: Prentice Hall, 1994.

23. Edington DW and Edgerton VR. *The Biology of Physical Activity*. Boston, MA: Houghton Mifflin, 1976.

24. Fleck S and Kraemer WJ. *Designing Resistance Training Programs*. Champaign, IL: Human Kinetics, 2004.

25. Fleck SJ and Kraemer WJ. *The Ultimate Training System: Periodization Breakthrough*. New York, NY: Advanced Research Press, 1996.

26. Foster C. Monitoring training in athletes with reference to overtraining syndrome. *Med Sci Sports Exerc* 30: 1164-1168, 1998.

27. Francis C. *Structure of Training for Speed*. charliefrancis.com, 2008, p 270.

28. Fry AC. The role of training intensity in resistance exercise overtraining and overreaching, in: *Overtraining in Sport*. RB Kreider, AC Fry, ML O'Toole, eds. Champaign, IL: Human Kinetics Publishers, 1998, pp 107-127.

29. Garcia-Pallares J, Garcia-Fernandez M, Sanchez-Medina L, and Izquierdo M. Performance changes in world-class kayakers following two different training periodization models. *Eur J Appl Physiol* 110: 99-107, 2010.

30. Gorostiaga EM, Navarro-Amezqueta I, Calbet JA, Hellsten Y, Cusso R, Guerrero M, Granados C, Gonzalez-Izal M, Ibanez J, and Izquierdo M. Energy metabolism during repeated sets of leg press exercise leading to failure or not. *PLoS One* 7: e40621, 2012.

31. Gourgoulis V, Aggeloussis N, Kasimatis P, Mavromatis G, and Garas A. Effect of a submaximal half-squats warm-up program on vertical jumping ability. *J Strength Cond Res* 17: 342-344, 2003.

32. Haff GG. Periodization of training. In *Conditioning for Strength and Human Performance*. LE Brown, J Chandler, eds. Philadelphia, PA: Wolters Kluwer, Lippincott, Williams & Wilkins, 2012, pp 326-345.

33. Haff GG. Peaking for competition in individual sports, in: *High-Performance Training for Sports*. D Joyce, D Lewindon, eds., Champaign, IL: Human Kinetics, 2014, pp 524-540.

34. Haff GG. Periodization strategies for youth development, in: *Strength and Conditioning for Young Athletes: Science and Application*. RS Lloyd, JL Oliver, eds. London: Routledge, Taylor & Francis Group, 2014, pp 149-168.

35. Haff GG, Burgess S, and Stone MH. Cluster training: theoretical and practical applications for the strength and conditioning professional. *Prof Strength and Cond* 12: 12-17, 2008.

36. Haff GG, Carlock JM, Hartman MJ, Kilgore JL, Kawamori N, Jackson JR, Morris RT, Sands WA, and Stone MH. Force-time curve characteristics of dynamic and isometric muscle actions of elite women Olympic weightlifters. *J Strength Cond Res* 19: 741-748, 2005.

37. Haff GG and Haff EE. Resistance training program design, in: *Essentials of Periodization*. MH Malek, JW Coburn, eds. Champaign, IL: Human Kinetics, 2012, pp 359-401.

38. Haff GG and Haff EE. Training integration and periodization. In *Strength and Conditioning Program Design*. J Hoffman, ed. Champaign, IL: Human Kinetics, 2012, pp 209-254.

39. Haff GG, Hobbs RT, Haff EE, Sands WA, Pierce KC, and Stone MH. Cluster training: a novel method for introducing training program variation. *Strength Cond J* 30: 67-76, 2008.

40. Haff GG and Nimphius S. Training principles for power. *Strength Cond J* 34: 2-12, 2012.

41. Haff GG, Ruben RP, Lider J, Twine C, and Cormie P. A comparison of methods for determining the rate of force development during isometric midthigh clean pulls. *J Strength Cond Res* 29: 386-395, 2015.

42. Haff GG, Stone MH, O'Bryant HS, Harman E, Dinan CN, Johnson R, and Han KH. Force-time dependent characteristics of dynamic and isometric muscle actions. *J Strength Cond Res* 11: 269-272, 1997.

43. Haff GG, Whitley A, and Potteiger JA. A brief review: explosive exercises and sports performance. *Natl Strength Cond Assoc* 23: 13-20, 2001.

44. Hardee JP, Travis Triplett N, Utter AC, Zwetsloot KA, and McBride JM. Effect of interrepetition rest on power output in the power clean. *J Strength Cond Res* 26: 883-889, 2012.

45. Harre D. *Principles of Sports Training*. Berlin, Germany: Democratic Republic: Sportverlag, 1982.

46. Harris GR, Stone MH, O'Bryant HS, Proulx CM, and Johnson RL. Short-term performance effects of high power, high force, or combined weight-training methods. *J Strength Cond Res* 14: 14-20, 2000.

47. Harris NK, Cronin JB, Hopkins WG, and Hansen KT. Squat jump training at maximal power loads vs. heavy loads: effect on sprint ability. *J Strength Cond Res* 22: 1742-1749, 2008.

48. Issurin V. Block periodization versus traditional training theory: a review. *J Sports Med Phys Fitness* 48: 65-75, 2008.

49. Issurin V. *Block Periodization: Breakthrough in Sports Training*. Michigan, USA: Ultimate Athlete Concepts, 2008.

50. Issurin VB. New horizons for the methodology and physiology of training periodization. *Sports Med* 40: 189-206, 2010.

51. Izquierdo M, Ibanez J, Gonzalez-Badillo JJ, Ratamess NA, Kraemer WJ, Häkkinen K, Bonnabau H, Granados C, French DN, and Gorostiaga EM. Detraining and tapering effects on hormonal responses and strength performance. *J Strength Cond Res* 21: 768-775, 2007.

52. Jeffreys I. Quadrennial planning for the high school athlete. *Strength Cond J* 30: 74-83, 2008.

53. Jovanović M. Planning the strength training. *Complementary Training.* Contemporary Training, 2009. http://complementarytraining.net/planning-the-strength-training-part-1/. Accessed February 9, 2017.

54. Kaneko M, Fuchimoto T, Toji H, and Suei K. Training effect of different loads on the force-velocity relationship and mechanical power output in human muscle. *Scand J Sports Sci* 5: 50-55, 1983.

55. Kawamori N and Haff GG. The optimal training load for the development of muscular power. *J Strength Cond Res* 18: 675-684, 2004.

56. Keiner M, Sander A, Wirth K, Caruso O, Immesberger P, and Zawieja M. Strength performance in youth: trainability of adolescents and children in the back and front squats. *J Strength Cond Res* 27: 357-362, 2013.

57. Kirby TJ, Erickson T, and McBride JM. Model for progression of strength, power, and speed training. *Strength Cond J* 32: 86-90 2010.

58. Knudson DV. Correcting the use of the term "power" in the strength and conditioning literature. *J Strength Cond Res* 23: 1902-1908, 2009.

59. Kraemer WJ and Fleck SJ. *Optimizing Strength Training: Designing Nonlinear Periodization Workouts.* Champaign, IL: Human Kinetics, 2007.

60. Kraemer WJ, Hatfield DL, and Fleck SJ. Types of muscle training, in: *Strength Training.* LE Brown, ed. Champaign, IL: Human Kinetics, 2007, pp 45-72.

61. Kurz T. *Science of Sports Training.* Island Pond, VT: Stadion Publishing Co., Inc., 2001.

62. Lovell DI, Cuneo R, and Gass GC. The effect of strength training and short-term detraining on maximum force and the rate of force development of older men. *Eur J Appl Physiol Occup Physiol* 109: 429-435, 2010.

63. Matveyev L. *Periodization of Sports Training.* Moskow, Russia: Fizkultura i Sport, 1965.

64. Matveyev LP. *Periodisterung Des Sportlichen Trainings.* Moscow: Fizkultura i Sport, 1972.

65. Matveyev LP. *Fundamentals of Sports Training.* Moscow: Fizkultua i Sport, 1977.

66. McBride JM, Nimphius S, and Erickson TM. The acute effects of heavy-load squats and loaded countermovement jumps on sprint performance. *J Strength Cond Res* 19: 893-897, 2005.

67. McBride JM, Triplett-McBride T, Davie A, and Newton RU. A comparison of strength and power characteristics between power lifters, Olympic lifters, and sprinters. *J Strength Cond Res* 13: 58-66, 1999.

68. McBride JM, Triplett-McBride T, Davie A, and Newton RU. The effect of heavy- vs. light-load jump squats on the development of strength, power, and speed. *J Strength Cond Res* 16: 75-82, 2002.

69. Minetti AE. On the mechanical power of joint extensions as affected by the change in muscle force (or cross-sectional area), ceteris paribus. *Eur J Appl Physiol* 86: 363-369, 2002.

70. Moss BM, Refsnes PE, Abildgaard A, Nicolaysen K, and Jensen J. Effects of maximal effort strength training with different loads on dynamic strength, cross-sectional area, load-power and load-velocity relationships. *Eur J Appl Physiol* 75: 193-199, 1997.

71. Mujika I and Padilla S. Detraining: loss of training-induced physiological and performance adaptations. Part I: short term insufficient training stimulus. *Sports Med* 30: 79-87, 2000.

72. Mujika I and Padilla S. Detraining: loss of training-induced physiological and performance adaptations. Part II: long term insufficient training stimulus. *Sports Med* 30: 145-154, 2000.

73. Mujika I and Padilla S. Scientific bases for precompetition tapering strategies. *Med Sci Sports Exerc* 35: 1182-1187, 2003.

74. Nádori L and Granek I. *Theoretical and Methodological Basis of Training Planning With Special Considerations Within a Microcycle.* Lincoln, NE: NSCA, 1989.

75. Newton RU and Kraemer WJ. Developing explosive muscular power: implications for a mixed methods training strategy. *Strength Cond J* 16: 20-31, 1994.

76. Olbrect J. *The Science of Winning: Planning, Periodizing, and Optimizing Swim Training.* Luton, England: Swimshop, 2000.

77. Painter KB, Haff GG, Ramsey MW, McBride J, Triplett T, Sands WA, Lamont HS, Stone ME, and Stone MH. Strength gains: block versus daily undulating periodization weight-training among track and field athletes. *Int J Sports Physiol Perform* 7: 161-169, 2012.

78. Plisk SS and Stone MH. Periodization strategies. *Strength and Cond* 25: 19-37, 2003.

79. Rhea MR, Ball SD, Phillips WT, and Burkett LN. A comparison of linear and daily undulating periodized programs with equated volume and intensity for strength. *Strength Cond J* 16: 250-255, 2002.

80. Roll F and Omer J. Football: Tulane football winter program. *Strength Cond J* 9: 34-38, 1987.

81. Rowbottom DG. Periodization of training, in: *Exercise and Sport Science*. WE Garrett, DT Kirkendall, eds. Philadelphia, PA: Lippicott Williams and Wilkins, 2000, pp 499-512.

82. Ruben RM, Molinari MA, Bibbee CA, Childress MA, Harman MS, Reed KP, and Haff GG. The acute effects of an ascending squat protocol on performance during horizontal plyometric jumps. *J Strength Cond Res* 24: 358-369, 2010.

83. Schmolinsky G. *Track and Field: The East German Textbook of Athletics*. Toronto, Canada: Sports Book Publisher, 2004.

84. Seitz L, Saez de Villarreal E, and Haff GG. The temporal profile of postactivation potentiation is related to strength level. *J Strength Cond Res* 28: 706-715, 2014.

85. Seitz LB and Haff GG. Application of methods of inducing postactivation potentiation during the preparation of rugby players. *Strength Cond J* 37: 40-49, 2015.

86. Seitz LB, Riviere M, de Villarreal ES, and Haff GG. The athletic performance of elite rugby league players is improved after an 8-week small-sided game training intervention. *J Strength Cond Res* 28: 971-975, 2014.

87. Seitz LB, Trajano GS, Dal Maso F, Haff GG, and Blazevich AJ. Postactivation potentiation during voluntary contractions after continued knee extensor task-specific practice. *Appl Physiol Nutr Metab* 40: 230-237, 2015.

88. Seitz LB, Trajano GS, and Haff GG. The back squat and the power clean elicit different degrees of potentiation. *Int J Sports Physiol Perform* 9: 643-649, 2014.

89. Selye H. *The Stress of Life*. New York, NY: McGraw-Hill, 1956.

90. Siff MC. *Supertraining*. Denver, CO: Supertraining Institute, 2003.

91. Smith DJ. A framework for understanding the training process leading to elite performance. *Sports Med* 33: 1103-1126, 2003.

92. Stone MH, Moir G, Glaister M, and Sanders R. How much strength is necessary? *Phys Ther Sport* 3: 88-96, 2002.

93. Stone MH, O'Bryant H, and Garhammer J. A hypothetical model for strength training. *J Sports Med* 21: 342-351, 1981.

94. Stone MH, Stone ME, and Sands WA. *Principles and Practice of Resistance Training*. Champaign, IL: Human Kinetics Publishers, 2007.

95. Sukop J and Nelson R. Effect of isometric training on the force-time characteristics of muscle contraction, in: *Biomechanics IV*. RC Nelson, CA Morehouse, eds. Baltimore, MD: University Park Press, 1974, pp 440-447.

96. Thibaudeau C. *Theory and Application of Modern Strength and Power Methods*. North Charleston, SC: Createspace Publishing, 2006.

97. Thorstensson A, Grimby G, and Karlsson J. Force-velocity relations and fiber composition in human knee extensor muscles. *J Appl Physiol* 40: 12-16, 1976.

98. Tillin NA and Bishop D. Factors modulating post-activation potentiation and its effect on performance of subsequent explosive activities. *Sports Med* 39: 147-166, 2009.

99. Toji H and Kaneko M. Effect of multiple-load training on the force-velocity relationship. *J Strength Cond Res* 18: 792-795, 2004.

100. Toji H, Suei K, and Kaneko M. Effects of combined training programs on force-velocity relation and power output in human muscle. *Jpn J Phys Fitness Sports Med* 44: 439-445, 1995.

101. Verkhoshansky Y and Siff MC. Application of special strength training means. In *Supertraining: Expanded Edition*. Rome, Italy: Verkoshansky, 2009, pp 287-294.

102. Verkhoshansky YU. How to set up a training program. *Sov Sports Rev* 16: 123-136, 1981.

103. Verkhoshansky YU. *Programming and Organization of Training*. Moscow: Fizkultura i Sport, 1985.

104. Verkhoshansky YU. *Fundamentals of Special Strength Training in Sport*. Livonia, MI: Sportivy Press, 1986.

105. Verkhoshansky YU. *Special Strength Training: A Practical Manual for Coaches.* Muskegon Heights, MI: Ultimate Athlete Concepts, 2006.

106. Verkhoshansky YU. Theory and methodology of sport preparation: block training system for top-level athletes. *Teoria i Practica Physicheskoj Culturi* 4: 2-14, 2007.

107. Verkoshansky Y and Siff MC. Programming and organisation of training. In *Supertraining: Expanded Editions*. Rome Italy: Verkoshansky, 2009, pp 313-392.

108. Viitasalo JT. Rate of force development, muscle structure and fatigue, in: *Biomechanics VII-A: Proceedings of the 7th International Congress of Biomechanics*. A Morecki, F Kazimirz, K Kedzior, A Wit, eds. Baltimore, MD: University Park Press, 1981, pp 136-141.

109. Wilson GJ, Newton RU, Murphy AJ, and Humphries BJ. The optimal training load for the development of dynamic athletic performance. *Med Sci Sports Exerc* 25: 1279-1286, 1993.

110. Yakovlev, N.N. *Sports Biochemistry.* Leipzig, Germany: Deutsche HochschuleKorperkulture (German Institute for Physical Culture), 1967.

111. Yetter M and Moir GL. The acute effects of heavy back and front squats on speed during forty-meter sprint trials. *J Strength Cond Res* 22: 159-165, 2008.

112. Zamparo P, Minetti AE, and di Prampero PE. Interplay among the changes of muscle strength, cross-sectional area and maximal explosive power: theory and facts. *Eur J Appl Physiol* 88: 193-202, 2002.

113. Zatsiorsky VM. Basic concepts of training theory. In *Science and Practice of Strength Training*. Champaign, IL: Human Kinetics, 1995, pp 3-19.

114. Zatsiorsky VM. Timing in strength training. In *Science and Practice of Strength Training*. Champaign, IL: Human Kinetics Publishers, 1995, pp 108-135.

115. Zatsiorsky VM and Kraemer WJ. *Science and Practice of Strength Training,* 2nd ed. Champaign, IL: Human Kinetics, 2006.

116. Zatsiorsky VM and Kraemer WJ. Timing in strength training. In *Science and Practice of Strength Training,* 2nd ed. Champaign, IL: Human Kinetics Publishes, 2006, pp 89-108.

Chapter 4

1. Arampatzis A, Degens H, Baltzopoulos V, and Rittweger J. Why do older sprinters reach the finish line later? *Exerc Sport Sci Rev* 39: 18-22, 2011.

2. Armstrong N, Welsman JR, and Chia MY. Short term power output in relation to growth and maturation. *Br J Sports Med* 35: 118-124, 2001.

3. Bean JF, Kiely DK, Herman S, Leveille SG, Mizer K, Frontera WR, and Fielding RA. The relationship between leg power and physical performance in mobility-limited older people. *J Am Geriatr Soc* 50: 461-467, 2002.

4. Behm DG and Sale DG. Intended rather than actual movement velocity determines velocity-specific training response. *J Appl Physiol* 74: 359-368, 1993.

5. Behringer M, Vom Heede A, Matthews M, and Mester J. Effects of strength training on motor performance skills in children and adolescents: a meta-analysis. *Pediatr Exerc Sci* 23: 186-206, 2011.

6. Beunen G and Malina RM. Growth and physical performance relative to the timing of the adolescent spurt. *Exerc Sport Sci Rev* 16: 503-540, 1988.

7. Beunen G, Ostyn M, Simons J, Renson R, Claessens AL, Vanden Eynde B, Lefevre J, Vanreusel B, Malina RM, and van't Hof MA. Development and tracking in fitness components: Leuven longitudinal study on lifestyle, fitness and health. *Int J Sports Med* 18 Suppl 3: S171-178, 1997.

8. Bonnefoy M, Kostka T, Arsac LM, Berthouze SE, and Lacour JR. Peak anaerobic power in elderly men. *Eur J Appl Physiol Occup Physiol* 77: 182-188, 1998.

9. Branta C, Haubenstricker J, and Seefeldt V. Age changes in motor skills during childhood and adolescence. *Exerc Sport Sci Rev* 12: 467-520, 1984.

10. Caserotti P, Aagaard P, Simonsen EB, and Puggaard L. Contraction-specific differences in maximal muscle power during stretch-shortening cycle movements in elderly males and females. *Eur J Appl Physiol* 84: 206-212, 2001.

11. Chaouachi A, Hammami R, Kaabi S, Chamari K, Drinkwater EJ, and Behm DG. Olympic weight-lifting and plyometric training with children provides similar or greater performance improvements than traditional resistance training. *J Strength Cond Res* 28: 1483-1496, 2014.

12. Cohen DD, Voss C, Taylor MJ, Delextrat A, Ogunleye AA, and Sandercock GR. Ten-year secular changes in muscular fitness in English children. *Acta Paediatr* 100: e175-177, 2011.

13. Cormie P, McGuigan MR, and Newton RU. Developing maximal neuromuscular power. Part II: training considerations for improving maximal power production. *Sports Med* 41: 125-146, 2011.

14. Cuoco A, Callahan DM, Sayers S, Frontera WR, Bean J, and Fielding RA. Impact of muscle power and force on gait speed in disabled older men and women. *J Gerontol A Biol Sci Med Sci* 59: 1200-1206, 2004.

15. Dayne AM, McBride JM, Nuzzo JL, Triplett NT, Skinner J, and Burr A. Power output in the jump squat in adolescent male athletes. *J Strength Cond Res* 25: 585-589, 2011.

16. de Vos NJ, Singh NA, Ross DA, Stavrinos TM, Orr R, and Fiatarone Singh MA. Optimal load for increasing muscle power during explosive resistance training in older adults. *J Gerontol A Biol Sci Med Sci* 60: 638-647, 2005.

17. de Vos NJ, Singh NA, Ross DA, Stavrinos TM, Orr R, and Fiatarone Singh MA. Effect of power-training intensity on the contribution of force and velocity to peak power in older adults. *J Aging Phys Act* 16: 393-407, 2008.

18. Dotan R, Mitchell C, Cohen R, Klentrou P, Gabriel D, and Falk B. Child-adult differences in muscle activation—a review. *Pediatr Exerc Sci* 24: 2-21, 2012.

19. Drey M, Sieber CC, Degens H, McPhee J, Korhonen MT, Muller K, Ganse B, and Rittweger J. Relation between muscle mass, motor units and type of training in master athletes. *Clin Physiol Funct Imaging* 36: 70-76, 2016.

20. Earles DR, Judge JO, and Gunnarsson OT. Velocity training induces power-specific adaptations in highly functioning older adults. *Arch Phys Med Rehabil* 82: 872-878, 2001.

21. Faigenbaum AD, Farrell A, Fabiano M, Radler T, Naclerio F, Ratamess NA, Kang J, and Myer GD. Effects of integrative neuromuscular training on fitness performance in children. *Pediatr Exerc Sci* 23: 573-584, 2011.

22. Faigenbaum AD, Farrell AC, Fabiano M, Radler TA, Naclerio F, Ratamess NA, Kang J, and Myer GD. Effects of detraining on fitness performance in 7-year-old children. *J Strength Cond Res* 27: 323-330, 2013.

23. Faigenbaum AD, Lloyd RS, and Myer GD. Youth resistance training: past practices, new perspectives, and future directions. *Pediatr Exerc Sci* 25: 591-604, 2013.

24. Fielding RA, LeBrasseur NK, Cuoco A, Bean J, Mizer K, and Fiatarone Singh MA. High-velocity resistance training increases skeletal muscle peak power in older women. *J Am Geriatr Soc* 50: 655-662, 2002.

25. Flanagan SD, Dunn-Lewis C, Hatfield DL, Distefano LJ, Fragala MS, Shoap M, Gotwald M, Trail J, Gomez AL, Volek JS, Cortis C, Comstock BA, Hooper DR, Szivak TK, Looney DP, DuPont WH, McDermott DM, Gaudiose MC, and Kraemer WJ. Developmental differences between boys and girls result in sex-specific physical fitness changes from fourth to fifth grade. *J Strength Cond Res* 29: 175-180, 2015.

26. Foldvari M, Clark M, Laviolette LC, Bernstein MA, Kaliton D, Castaneda C, Pu CT, Hausdorff JM, Fielding RA, and Singh MA. Association of muscle power with functional status in community-dwelling elderly women. *J Gerontol A Biol Sci Med Sci* 55: M192-199, 2000.

27. Ford KR, Myer GD, Brent JL, and Hewett TE. Hip and knee extensor moments predict vertical jump height in adolescent girls. *J Strength Cond Res* 23: 1327-1331, 2009.

28. Gorostiaga EM, Izquierdo M, Ruesta M, Iribarren J, Gonzalez-Badillo JJ, and Ibanez J. Strength training effects on physical performance and serum hormones in young soccer players. *Eur J Appl Physiol* 91: 698-707, 2004.

29. Hakkinen K, Kraemer WJ, Newton RU, and Alen M. Changes in electromyographic activity, muscle fibre and force production characteristics during heavy resistance/power strength training in middle-aged and older men and women. *Acta Physiol Scand* 171: 51-62, 2001.

30. Harries SK, Lubans DR, and Callister R. Resistance training to improve power and sports performance in adolescent athletes: a systematic review and meta-analysis. *J Sci Med Sport* 15: 532-540, 2012.

31. Harrison AJ and Gaffney S. Motor development and gender effects on stretch-shortening cycle performance. *J Sci Med Sport* 4: 406-415, 2001.

32. Hazell T, Kenno K, and Jakobi J. Functional benefit of power training for older adults. *J Aging Phys Act* 15: 349-359, 2007.

33. Hinman JD, Peters A, Cabral H, Rosene DL, Hollander W, Rasband MN, and Abraham CR. Age-related molecular reorganization at the node of Ranvier. *J Comp Neurol* 495: 351-362, 2006.

34. Jankelowitz SK, McNulty PA, and Burke D. Changes in measures of motor axon excitability with age. *Clin Neurophysiol* 118: 1397-1404, 2007.

35. Keiner M, Sander A, Wirth K, Caruso O, Immesberger P, and Zawieja M. Strength performance in youth: trainability of adolescents and children in the back and front squats. *J Strength Cond Res* 27: 357-362, 2013.

36. Komi PV. Stretch-shortening cycle: a powerful model to study normal and fatigued muscle. *J Biomech* 33: 1197-1206, 2000.

37. Leard JS, Cirillo MA, Katsnelson E, Kimiatek DA, Miller TW, Trebincevic K, and Garbalosa JC. Validity of two alternative systems for measuring vertical jump height. *J Strength Cond Res* 21: 1296-1299, 2007.

38. Lexell J. Ageing and human muscle: observations from Sweden. *Can J Appl Physiol* 18: 2-18, 1993.

39. Lloyd RS, Cronin JB, Faigenbaum AD, Haff GG, Howard R, Kraemer WJ, Micheli LJ, Myer GD, and Oliver JL. The National Strength and Conditioning Association position statement on long-term athletic development. *J Strength Cond Res* 30: 1491-1509, 2016.

40. Lloyd RS, Faigenbaum AD, Stone MH, Oliver JL, Jeffreys I, Moody JA, Brewer C, Pierce KC, McCambridge TM, Howard R, Herrington L, Hainline B, Micheli LJ, Jaques R, Kraemer WJ, McBride MG, Best TM, Chu DA, Alvar BA, and Myer GD. Position statement on youth resistance training: the 2014 International Consensus. *Br J Sports Med* 48: 498-505, 2014.

41. Lloyd RS and Oliver JL. The youth physical development model: a new approach to long-term athletic development. *Strength Cond J* 34: 61-72, 2012.

42. Lloyd RS, Oliver JL, Faigenbaum AD, Myer GD, and De Ste Croix MB. Chronological age vs. biological maturation: implications for exercise programming in youth. *J Strength Cond Res* 28: 1454-1464, 2014.

43. Lloyd RS, Oliver JL, Hughes MG, and Williams CA. Reliability and validity of field-based measures of leg stiffness and reactive strength index in youths. *J Sports Sci* 27: 1565-1573, 2009.

44. Lloyd RS, Oliver JL, Hughes MG, and Williams CA. The influence of chronological age on periods of accelerated adaptation of stretch-shortening cycle performance in pre and postpubescent boys. *J Strength Cond Res* 25: 1889-1897, 2011.

45. Lloyd RS, Oliver JL, Hughes MG, and Williams CA. Specificity of test selection for the appropriate assessment of different measures of stretch-shortening cycle function in children. *J Sports Med Phys Fitness* 51: 595-602, 2011.

46. Lloyd RS, Oliver JL, Hughes MG, and Williams CA. Age-related differences in the neural regulation of stretch-shortening cycle activities in male youths during maximal and sub-maximal hopping. *J Electromyogr Kinesiol* 22: 37-43, 2012.

47. Lloyd RS, Oliver JL, Hughes MG, and Williams CA. The effects of 4-weeks of plyometric training on reactive strength index and leg stiffness in male youths. *J Strength Cond Res* 26: 2812-2819, 2012.

48. Malina RM, Eisenmann JC, Cumming SP, Ribeiro B, and Aroso J. Maturity-associated variation in the growth and functional capacities of youth football (soccer) players 13-15 years. *Eur J Appl Physiol* 91: 555-562, 2004.

49. Marsh AP, Miller ME, Rejeski WJ, Hutton SL, and Kritchevsky SB. Lower extremity muscle function after strength or power training in older adults. *J Aging Phys Act* 17: 416-443, 2009.

50. Matos N and Winsley RJ. Trainability of young athletes and overtraining. *J Sports Sci Med* 6: 353-367, 2007.

51. McMaster DT, Gill N, Cronin J, and McGuigan M. A brief review of strength and ballistic assessment methodologies in sport. *Sports Med* 44: 603-623, 2014.

52. Meylan CM, Cronin JB, Oliver JL, Hopkins WG, and Contreras B. The effect of maturation on adaptations to strength training and detraining in 11-15-year-olds. *Scand J Med Sci Sports* 24: e156-164, 2014.

53. Meylan CMP, Cronin JB, Oliver JL, Hughes MG, and Manson S. An evidence-based model of power development in youth soccer. *J Sports Sci Coaching* 9: 1241-1264, 2014.

54. Miszko TA, Cress ME, Slade JM, Covey CJ, Agrawal SK, and Doerr CE. Effect of strength and power training on physical function in community-dwelling older adults. *J Gerontol A Biol Sci Med Sci* 58: 171-175, 2003.

55. Myer GD, Lloyd RS, Brent JL, and Faigenbaum AD. How young is "too young" to start training? *ACSMs Health Fit J* 17: 14-23, 2013.

56. Newton RU, Hakkinen K, Hakkinen A, McCormick M, Volek J, and Kraemer WJ. Mixed-methods resistance training increases power and strength of young and older men. *Med Sci Sports Exerc* 34: 1367-1375, 2002.

57. Newton RU and Kraemer WJ. Developing explosive power: implications for a mixed method training strategy. *Strength Cond J* 16: 20-31, 1994.

58. Nogueira W, Gentil P, Mello SN, Oliveira RJ, Bezerra AJ, and Bottaro M. Effects of power training on muscle thickness of older men. *Int J Sports Med* 30: 200-204, 2009.

59. Pereira A, Izquierdo M, Silva AJ, Costa AM, Bastos E, Gonzalez-Badillo JJ, and Marques MC. Effects of high-speed power training on functional capacity and muscle performance in older women. *Exp Gerontol* 47: 250-255, 2012.

60. Pescatello LS, Arena R, Riebe D, and Thompson PD. *ACSM's Guidelines for Exercise Testing and Prescription*. Philadelphia, PA: Lippincott, Willliams, and Wilkins, 2014.

61. Petrella JK, Kim JS, Tuggle SC, and Bamman MM. Contributions of force and velocity to improved power with progressive resistance training in young and older adults. *Eur J Appl Physiol* 99: 343-351, 2007.

62. Piirainen JM, Cronin NJ, Avela J, and Linnamo V. Effects of plyometric and pneumatic explosive strength training on neuromuscular function and dynamic balance control in 60-70 year old males. *J Electromyogr Kinesiol* 24: 246-252, 2014.

63. Porter MM. Power training for older adults. *Appl Physiol Nutr Metab* 31: 87-94, 2006.

64. Porter MM, Vandervoort AA, and Lexell J. Aging of human muscle: structure, function and adaptability. *Scand J Med Sci Sports* 5: 129-142, 1995.

65. Quatman CE, Ford KR, Myer GD, and Hewett TE. Maturation leads to gender differences in landing force and vertical jump performance: a longitudinal study. *Am J Sports Med* 34: 806-813, 2006.

66. Regterschot GR, Zhang W, Baldus H, Stevens M, and Zijlstra W. Sensor-based monitoring of sit-to-stand performance is indicative of objective and self-reported aspects of functional status in older adults. *Gait Posture* 41: 935-940, 2015.

67. Reid KF and Fielding RA. Skeletal muscle power: a critical determinant of physical functioning in older adults. *Exerc Sport Sci Rev* 40: 4-12, 2012.

68. Reid KF, Martin KI, Doros G, Clark DJ, Hau C, Patten C, Phillips EM, Frontera WR, and Fielding RA. Comparative effects of light or heavy resistance power training for improving lower extremity power and physical performance in mobility-limited older adults. *J Gerontol A Biol Sci Med Sci* 70: 374-380, 2015.

69. Reilly T, Williams AM, Nevill A, and Franks A. A multidisciplinary approach to talent identification in soccer. *J Sports Sci* 18: 695-702, 2000.

70. Runhaar J, Collard DC, Singh AS, Kemper HC, van Mechelen W, and Chinapaw M. Motor fitness in Dutch youth: differences over a 26-year period (1980-2006). *J Sci Med Sport* 13: 323-328, 2010.

71. Sander A, Keiner M, Wirth K, and Schmidtbleicher D. Influence of a 2-year strength training programme on power performance in elite youth soccer players. *Eur J Sport Sci* 13: 445-451, 2013.

72. Sayers SP, Bean J, Cuoco A, LeBrasseur NK, Jette A, and Fielding RA. Changes in function and disability after resistance training: does velocity matter? a pilot study. *Am J Phys Med Rehabil* 82: 605-613, 2003.

73. Sayers SP and Gibson K. A comparison of high-speed power training and traditional slow-speed resistance training in older men and women. *J Strength Cond Res* 24: 3369-3380, 2010.

74. Shaibi GQ, Cruz ML, Ball GD, Weigensberg MJ, Salem GJ, Crespo NC, and Goran MI. Effects of resistance training on insulin sensitivity in overweight Latino adolescent males. *Med Sci Sports Exerc* 38: 1208-1215, 2006.

75. Skelton DA, Greig CA, Davies JM, and Young A. Strength, power and related functional ability of healthy people aged 65-89 years. *Age Ageing* 23: 371-377, 1994.

76. Skelton DA, Kennedy J, and Rutherford OM. Explosive power and asymmetry in leg muscle function in frequent fallers and non-fallers aged over 65. *Age Ageing* 31: 119-125, 2002.

77. Stone MH, O'Bryant HS, McCoy L, Coglianese R, Lehmkuhl M, and Schilling B. Power and maximum strength relationships during performance of dynamic and static weighted jumps. *J Strength Cond Res* 17: 140-147, 2003.

78. Tonson A, Ratel S, Le Fur Y, Cozzone P, and Bendahan D. Effect of maturation on the relationship between muscle size and force production. *Med Sci Sports Exerc* 40: 918-925, 2008.

79. Tremblay MS, Gray CE, Akinroye K, Harrington DM, Katzmarzyk PT, Lambert EV, Liukkonen J, Maddison R, Ocansey RT, Onywera VO, Prista A, Reilly JJ, Rodriguez Martinez MP, Sarmiento Duenas OL, Standage M, and Tomkinson G. Physical activity of children: a global matrix of grades comparing 15 countries. *J Phys Act Health* 11 Suppl 1: S113-125, 2014.

80. Tschopp M, Sattelmayer MK, and Hilfiker R. Is power training or conventional resistance training better for function in elderly persons? A meta-analysis. *Age Ageing* 40: 549-556, 2011.

81. Tudorascu I, Sfredel V, Riza AL, Danciulescu Miulescu R, Ianosi SL, and Danoiu S. Motor unit changes in normal aging: a brief review. *Rom J Morphol Embryol* 55: 1295-1301, 2014.

82. Ward RE, Boudreau RM, Caserotti P, Harris TB, Zivkovic S, Goodpaster BH, Satterfield S, Kritchevsky S, Schwartz AV, Vinik AI, Cauley JA, Newman AB, Strotmeyer ES, and Health ABC Study. Sensory and motor peripheral nerve function and longitudinal changes in quadriceps strength. *J Gerontol A Biol Sci Med Sci* 70: 464-470, 2015.

83. Wong PL, Chamari K, and Wisloff U. Effects of 12-week on-field combined strength and power training on physical performance among U-14 young soccer players. *J Strength Cond Res* 24: 644-652, 2010.

Chapter 5

1. Argus CK, Gill ND, Keogh JW, and Hopkins WG. Assessing the variation in the load that produces maximal upper-body power. *J Strength Cond Res* 28: 240-244, 2014.

2. Baker D. A series of studies on the training of high-intensity muscle power in rugby league football players. *J Strength Cond Res* 15: 198-209, 2001.

3. Baker D, Nance S, and Moore M. The load that maximizes the average mechanical power output during explosive bench press throws in highly trained athletes. *J Strength Cond Res* 15: 20-24, 2001.

4. Bartolomei S, Hoffman JR, Merni F, and Stout JR. A comparison of traditional and block periodized strength training programs in trained athletes. *J Strength Cond Res* 28: 990-997, 2014.

5. Bellar DM, Muller MD, Barkley JE, Kim CH, Ida K, Ryan EJ, Bliss MV, and Glickman EL. The effects of combined elastic- and free-weight tension vs. free-weight tension on one-repetition maximum strength in the bench press. *J Strength Cond Res* 25: 459-463, 2011.

6. Bevan HR, Bunce PJ, Owen NJ, Bennett MA, Cook CJ, Cunningham DJ, Newton RU, and Kilduff LP. Optimal loading for the development of peak power output in professional rugby players. *J Strength Cond Res* 24: 43-47, 2010.

7. Bouhlel E, Chelly MS, Tabka Z, and Shephard R. Relationships between maximal anaerobic power of the arms and legs and javelin performance. *J Sports Med Phys Fitness* 47: 141-146, 2007.

8. Calatayud J, Borreani S, Colado JC, Martin F, Tella V, and Andersen LL. Bench press and push-up at comparable levels of muscle activity results in similar strength gains. *J Strength Cond Res* 29: 246-253, 2015.

9. Chelly MS, Hermassi S, Aouadi R, and Shephard RJ. Effects of 8-week in-season plyometric training on upper and lower limb performance of elite adolescent handball players. *J Strength Cond Res* 28: 1401-1410, 2014.

10. Chelly MS, Hermassi S, and Shephard RJ. Relationships between power and strength of the upper and lower limb muscles and throwing velocity in male handball players. *J Strength Cond Res* 24: 1480-1487, 2010.

11. Comstock BA, Solomon-Hill G, Flanagan SD, Earp JE, Luk HY, Dobbins KA, Dunn-Lewis C, Fragala MS, Ho JY, Hatfield DL, Vingren JL, Denegar CR, Volek JS, Kupchak BR, Maresh CM, and Kraemer WJ. Validity of the Myotest in measuring force and power production in the squat and bench press. *J Strength Cond Res* 25: 2293-2297, 2011.

12. Dines JS, Bedi A, Williams PN, Dodson CC, Ellenbecker TS, Altchek DW, Windler G, and Dines DM. Tennis injuries: epidemiology, pathophysiology, and treatment. *J Am Acad Orthop Surg* 23: 181-189, 2015.

13. Dunn-Lewis C, Luk HY, Comstock BA, Szivak TK, Hooper DR, Kupchak BR, Watts AM, Putney BJ, Hydren JR, Volek JS, Denegar CR, and Kraemer WJ. The effects of a customized over-the-counter mouth guard on neuromuscular force and power production in trained men and women. *J Strength Cond Res* 26: 1085-1093, 2012.

14. Durall CJ, Udermann BE, Johansen DR, Gibson B, Reineke DM, and Reuteman P. The effects of preseason trunk muscle training on low-back pain occurrence in women collegiate gymnasts. *J Strength Cond Res* 23: 86-92, 2009.

15. Earp JE and Kraemer WJ. Medicine ball training implications for rotational power sports. *Strength Cond J* 32: 20-25, 2010.

16. Falvo MJ, Schilling BK, and Weiss LW. Techniques and considerations for determining isoinertial upper-body power. *Sports Biomech* 5: 293-311, 2015.

17. Ghigiarelli JJ, Nagle EF, Gross FL, Robertson RJ, Irrgang JJ, and Myslinski T. The effects of a 7-week heavy elastic band and weight chain program on upper-body strength and upper-body power in a sample of division 1-AA football players. *J Strength Cond Res* 23: 756-764, 2009.

18. Goto K and Morishima T. Compression garment promotes muscular strength recovery after resistance exercise. *Med Sci Sports Exerc* 46: 2265-2270, 2014.

19. Hooper DR, Dulkis LL, Secola PJ, Holtzum G, Harper SP, Kalkowski RJ, Comstock BA, Szivak TK, Flanagan SD, Looney DP, DuPont WH, Maresh CM, Volek JS, Culley KP, and Kraemer WJ. The roles of an upper body compression garment on athletic performances. *J Strength Cond Res*, 29: 2655-2660, 2015.

20. Jancosko JJ and Kazanjian JE. Shoulder injuries in the throwing athlete. *Phys Sportsmed* 40: 84-90, 2012.

21. Jones MT. Effect of compensatory acceleration training in combination with accommodating resistance on upper body strength in collegiate athletes. *Open Access J Sports Med* 5: 183-189, 2014.

22. Joy JM, Lowery RP, Oliveira de Souza E, and Wilson JM. Elastic bands as a component of periodized resistance training. *J Strength Cond Res*, 30: 2100-2106, 2016.

23. Kennedy DJ, Visco CJ, and Press J. Current concepts for shoulder training in the overhead athlete. *Curr Sports Med Rep* 8: 154-160, 2009.

24. Kibler WB, Press J, and Sciascia A. The role of core stability in athletic function. *Sports Med* 36: 189-198, 2006.

25. Kraemer WJ, Flanagan SD, Comstock BA, Fragala MS, Earp JE, Dunn-Lewis C, Ho JY, Thomas GA, Solomon-Hill G, Penwell ZR, Powell MD, Wolf MR, Volek JS, Denegar CR, and Maresh CM. Effects of a whole body compression garment on markers of recovery after a heavy resistance workout in men and women. *J Strength Cond Res* 24: 804-814, 2010.

26. Mayhew JL, Johns RA, and Ware JS. Changes in absolute upper body power following resistance training in college males. *J Appl Sport Science Res*: 187, 1992.

27. McGill SM. Low back stability: from formal description to issues for performance and rehabilitation. *Exerc Sport Sci Rev* 29: 26-31, 2001.

28. McGill SM, Childs A, and Liebenson C. Endurance times for low back stabilization exercises: clinical targets for testing and training from a normal database. *Arch Phys Med Rehabil* 80: 941-944, 1999.

29. Newton RU, Murphy AJ, Humphries BJ, Wilson GJ, Kraemer WJ, and Hakkinen K. Influence of load and stretch shortening cycle on the kinematics, kinetics and muscle activation that occurs during explosive upper-body movements. *Eur J Appl Physiol Occup Physiol* 75: 333-342, 1997.

30. Rucci JA and Tomporowski PD. Three types of kinematic feedback and the execution of the hang power clean. *J Strength Cond Res* 24: 771-778, 2010.

31. Shinkle J, Nesser TW, Demchak TJ, and McMannus DM. Effect of core strength on the measure of power in the extremities. *J Strength Cond Res* 26: 373-380, 2012.

32. Shoepe TC, Ramirez DA, Rovetti RJ, Kohler DR, and Almstedt HC. The effects of 24 weeks of resistance training with simultaneous elastic and free weight loading on muscular performance of novice lifters. *J Hum Kinet* 29: 93-106, 2011.

Chapter 7

1. Baker D and Nance S. The relation between running speed and measures of strength and power in professional rugby league players. *J Strength Cond Res* 13: 230-235, 1999.

2. Canavan PK, Garrett GE, and Armstrong LE. Kinematic and kinetic relationships between an Olympic-style lift and the vertical jump. *J Strength Cond Res* 10: 127-130, 1996.

3. Carlock JM, Smith SL, Hartman MJ, Morris RT, Ciroslan DA, Pierce KC, Newton RU, Harman EA, Sands WA, and Stone MH. The relationship between vertical jump power estimates and weightlifting ability: a field-test approach. *J Strength Cond Res* 18: 534-539, 2004.

4. Channell BT and Barfield JP. Effect of Olympic and traditional resistance training on vertical jump improvement in high school boys. *J Strength Cond Res* 22: 1522–1527, 2008.

5. Cormie P, McCaulley G, Triplett N, and McBride J. Optimal loading for maximal power output during lower-body resistance exercises. *Med Sci Sports Exerc* 39: 340-349, 2007.

6. Cormie P, McGuigan MR, and Newton RU. Developing maximal neuromuscular power. Part I: biological basis of maximal power production. *Sports Med* 41: 17-38, 2011a.

7. Cormie P, McGuigan MR, and Newton RU. Developing maximal neuromuscular power. Part II: training considerations for improving maximal power production. *Sports Med* 41: 125-146, 2011b.

8. Garhammer J. Power production by Olympic weightlifters. *Med Sci Sports Exerc* 12: 54-60, 1980.

9. Garhammer J. Energy flow during Olympic weightlifting. *Med Sci Sports Exerc* 14: 353-360, 1982.

10. Garhammer J. A comparison of maximal power outputs between elite male and female weightlifters in competition. *Int J Sport Biomech* 7: 3-11, 1991.

11. Garhammer J. A review of power output studies of Olympic and powerlifting: methodology, performance prediction, and evaluation tests. *J Strength Cond Res* 7: 76-89, 1993.

12. Garhammer J and Gregor R. Propulsion forces as a function of intensity for weightlifting and vertical jumping. *J Appl Sports Sci Res* 6: 129–134, 1992.

13. Hori N, Newton RU, Andrews WA, Kawamori N, McGuigan MR, and Nosaka K. Does performance of hang power clean differentiate performance of jumping, sprinting, and changing of direction? *J Strength Cond Res* 22: 412-418, 2008.

14. Kawamori N, Crum AJ, Blumert PA, Kulik JR, Childers JT, Wood JA, Stone MH, and Haff GG. Influence of different relative intensities on power output during the hang power clean: identification of the optimal load. *J Strength Cond Res* 19: 698-708, 2005.

15. Kilduff L, Bevan H, Owen N, Kingsley M, Bunce P, Bennett M, and Cunningham D. Optimal loading for peak power output during the hang power clean in professional rugby players. *Int J Sports Physiol Perform* 2: 260-269, 2007.

16. Storey A and Smith H. Unique aspects of competitive weightlifting: performance, training and physiology. *Sports Med* 42: 769-790, 2012.

17. Tricoli V, Lamas L, Carnevale R, and Ugrinowitsch C. Short-term effects on lower-body functional power development: weightlifting vs. vertical jump training programs. *J Strength Cond Res* 19: 433-437, 2005.

Chapter 8

1. Adams K, O'Shea J, O'Shea K, and Climstein M. The effects of six weeks of squat, plyometric and squat-plyometric training on power production. *J Appl Sport Sci Res* 6: 36-41, 1992.

2. Anderson C, Sforzo G, and Sigg J. The effects of combining elastic and free weight resistance on strength and power in athletes. *J Strength Cond Res* 22: 567-574, 2008.

3. Baker D. A series of studies on the training of high intensity muscle power in rugby league football players. *J Strength Cond Res* 15: 198-209, 2001.

4. Baker D and Nance S. The relationship between strength and power in professional rugby league players. *J Strength Cond Res* 13: 224-229, 1999.

5. Baker D and Newton R. Methods to increase the effectiveness of maximal power training for the upper body. *J Strength Cond Res* 27: 24-32, 2005.

6. Baker D and Newton R. Effect of kinetically altering a repetition via the use of chain resistance on velocity during the bench press. *J Strength Cond Res* 23: 1941-1946, 2009.

7. Bellar D, Muller M, Barkley J, Kim C, Ida K, Ryan E, Bliss M, and Glickman E. The effects of combined elastic- and free-weight tension vs. free-weight tension on one-repetition maximum strength in the bench press. *J Strength Cond Res* 25: 459-463, 2011.

8. Berning J, Coker C, and Adams K. Using chains for strength and conditioning. *Strength and Cond J* 26: 80-84, 2004.

9. Blazevich A, Gill N, Bronks R, and Newton R. Training-specific muscle architecture adaptation after 5-wk training in athletes. *Med Sci Sports Exerc* 35: 2013-2022, 2003.

10. Brandon R, Howatson G, Strachan F, and Hunter A. Neuromuscular response differences to power vs strength back squat exercise in elite athletes. *Scand J Med Sci Sport* 25: 630-639, 2015.

11. Burger T, Boyer-Kendrick T, and Dolny D. Complex training compared to a combined weight training and plyometric training program. *J Strength Cond Res* 14: 360, 2000.

12. Carlock J, Smith S, Hartman M, Morris R, Ciroslan D, Pierce K, Newton R, Hartman E, Sands W, and Stone M. The relationship between vertical jump power estimates and weightlifting ability: a field-test approach. *J Strength Cond Res* 18: 534-539, 2004.

13. Chatzopoulos D, Michailidis C, Giannakos A, Alexiou K, Patikas D, Antonopoulos C, and Kotzamanidis C. Postactivation potentiation effects after heavy resistance exercise on running speed. *J Strength Cond Res* 21: 1278-1281, 2007.

14. Chiu L, Fry A, Schilling B, Johnson E, and Weiss L. Neuromuscular fatigue and potentiation following two successive high intensity resistance exercise sessions. *Eur J Appl Physiol Occup Physiol* 92: 385-392, 2004.

15. Chiu L, Fry A, Weiss L, Schilling B, Brown L, and Smith S. Postactivation potentiation response in athletic and recreationally trained individuals. *J Strength Cond Res* 17: 671-677, 2003.

16. Clark R, Bryant A, and Humphries B. A comparison of force curve profiles between the bench press and ballistic bench throws. *J Strength Cond Res* 22: 1755-1759, 2008.

17. Cormie P, McGuigan M, and Newton R. Influence of strength on magnitude and mechanisms of adaptation to power training. *Med Sci Sports Exerc* 42: 1566-1581, 2010.

18. Cormie P, McGuigan M, and Newton R. Developing maximal neuromuscular power. Part II: training considerations for improved maximal power production. *Sports Med* 41: 125-146, 2011.

19. Cormie P, McGuigan M, and Newton R. Developing neuromuscular power. Part I: biological basis of maximal power production. *Sports Med* 41: 17-38, 2011.

20. Cronin J, McNair P, and Marshall R. The effects of bungee weight training on muscle function and functional performance. *J Sport Sci* 21: 59-71, 2003.

21. Cronin J, McNair P, and Marshall R. Force–velocity analysis of strength-training techniques and load: implications for training strategy and research. *J Strength Cond Res* 17: 148-155, 2003.

22. Dapena J. The high jump, in: *Biomechanics in Sport: Performance Enhancement and Injury Prevention.* Zatsiorsky V, ed. Oxford, UK: Blackwell Science, 2000, pp 284-311.

23. de Villarreal E, Izquierdo M, and Gonzalez-Badillo J. Enhancing jumping performance after combined vs. maximal power, heavy-resistance, and plyometric training alone. *J Strength Cond Res* 25: 3274-3281, 2011.

24. Docherty D and Hodgson M. The application of postactivation potentiation to elite sport. *Int J Sports Physiol Perf* 2: 439-444, 2007.

25. Ebben W. Complex training: a brief review. *J Sport Sci Med* 1: 42-46, 2002.

26. Ebben W and Jensen R. Electromyographic and kinematic analysis of traditional, chain, and elastic band squats. *J Strength Cond Res* 16: 547-550, 2002.

27. Ebben W and Watts P. A review of combined weight training and plyometric training modes: complex training. *Strength and Cond J* 20: 18-27, 1998.

28. Elliot B, Wilson G, and Kerr G. A biomechanical analysis of the sticking region in the bench press. *Med Sci Sports Exerc* 21: 450-462, 1989.

29. Evans A, Hodgkins T, Durham M, Berning J, and Adams K. The acute effects of 5RM bench press on power output. *Med Sci Sports Exerc* 32: S311, 2000.

30. Faigenbaum A, O'Connell J, La Rosa R, and Westcott W. Effects of strength training and complex training on upper-body strength and endurance development in children. *J Strength Cond Res* 13: 424, 1999.

31. Fatourous I, Jamurtas A, Leontsini D, Taxildaris K, Aggelousis N, Kostopoulos N, and Buckenmeyer P. Evaluation of plyometric exercise training, weight training, and their combination on vertical jump and leg strength. *J Strength Cond Res* 14: 470-476, 2000.

32. Flanagan E and Comyns T. The use of contact time and the reactive strength index to optimize fast stretch-shortening cycle training. *Strength and Cond J* 30: 33-38, 2008.

33. Fleck S and Kraemer W. *Designing Resistance Training Programs*. Champaign, IL: Human Kinetics, 2004.

34. Folland J and Williams A. The adaptations to strength training: morphological and neurological contributions to increased strength. *Sports Med* 37: 145-168, 2007.

35. French D, Kraemer W, and Cooke C. Changes in dynamic exercise performance following a sequence of preconditioning isometric muscle actions. *J Strength Cond Res* 17: 678-685, 2003.

36. Friedmann-Bette B, Bauer T, Kinscherf R, Vorwald S, Klute K, Bischoff D, Müller H, Weber M, Metz J, Kauczor H, Bärtsch P, and Billeter R. Effects of strength training with eccentric overload on muscle adaptation in male athletes. *Sports Med* 108: 821-836, 2010.

37. Frost D, Cronin J, and Newton R. A biomechanical evaluation of resistance: fundamental concepts for training and sports performance. *Sports Med* 40: 303-326, 2010.

38. García-Ramos A, Padial P, Haff G, Argüelles-Cienfuegos J, García-Ramos M, Conde-Pipó J, and Feriche B. Effect of different interrepetition rest periods on barbell velocity loss during the ballistic bench press exercise. *J Strength Cond Res* 29: 2388-2396, 2015.

39. Garhammer J. A review of power output studies of Olympic and powerlifting: methodology, performance prediction, and evaluation tests. *J Strength Cond Res* 7: 76-89, 1993.

40. Gilbert G, Lees A, and Graham-Smith P. Temporal profile of post-tetanic potentiation of muscle force characteristics after repeated maximal exercise. *J Sport Sci* 19: 6, 2001.

41. Gonzalez-Badillo J and Sanchez-Medina L. Movement velocity as a measure of loading intensity in resistance training. *Int J Sports Med* 31: 347-352, 2010.

42. Gourgoulis V, Aggeloussis N, Kasimatis P, Mavromatis G, and Garas A. Effect of a submaximal half-squats warm-up program on vertical jumping ability. *J Strength Cond Res* 17: 342-344, 2003.

43. Gullich A and Schmidtbleicher D. MVC-induced short-term potentiation of explosive force. *N Stud Athlet* 11: 67-81, 1996.

44. Haff G, Burgess S, and Stone M. Cluster training: theoretical and practical applications for the strength and conditioning professional. *Prof Strength Cond* 12: 12-16, 2008.

45. Haff G, Whitley A, McCoy L, O'Bryant H, Kilgore J, Haff E, Pierce K, and Stone M. Effects of different set configurations on barbell velocity and displacement during clean pull. *J Strength Cond Res* 17: 95-103, 2003.

46. Hamada T, Sale D, MacDougall J, and Tarnopolsky MA. Interaction of fibre type, potentiation and fatigue in human knee extensor muscles. *Acta Physiol Scand* 178: 165-173, 2003.

47. Hodgson M, Docherty D, and Robbins D. Post-activation potentiation: underlying physiology and implications for motor performance. *Sports Med* 35: 585-595, 2005.

48. Hori N, Newton R, Nosaka K, and Stone M. Weightlifting exercises enhance athletic performance that requires high-load speed strength. *Strength and Cond J* 27: 50-55, 2005.

49. Israetel M, McBride J, Nuzzo J, Skinner J, and Dayne A. Kinetic and kinematic differences between squats performed with and without elastic bands. *J Strength Cond Res* 24: 190-194, 2010.

50. Jandacka D and Beremlijski P. Determination of strength exercise intensities based on the load-power-velocity relationship. *J Hum Kinetics* 28: 33-44, 2011.

51. Jeffreys I. A review of post activation potentiation and its application in strength and conditioning. *Prof Strength Cond* 12: 17-25, 2008.

52. Jidovtseff B, Quievre J, Hanon C, and Crielaard J. Inertial muscular profiles allow a more accurate training load definition. *Sci and Sports* 24: 91-96, 2009.

53. Joy J, Lowery P, Oliveira De Souza E, and Wilson J. Elastic bands as a component of periodized resistance training. *J Strength Cond Res* 30: 2100-2106, 2016. .

54. Kaneko M, Fuchimoto T, Toji H, and Suei K. Training effects of different loads on the force-velocity relationship and mechanical power output in human muscle. *Scand J Sport Sci* 5: 50-55, 1983.

55. Kawamori N and Haff G. The optimal training load for the development of muscular power. *J Strength Cond Res* 18: 675-684, 2004.

56. Kilduff L, Bevan H, Kingsley M, Owen N, Bennett M, Bunce P, Hore A, Maw J, and Cunningham D. Postactivation potentiation in professional rugby players: optimal recovery. *J Strength Cond Res* 21: 1134-1138, 2007.

57. Knudson D. Correcting the use of the term "power" in the strength and conditioning literature. *J Strength Cond Res* 23: 1902-1908, 2009.

58. Komi P and Virmavirta M. Determinants of successful ski-jumping performance, in: *Biomechanics in Sport: Performance Enhancement and Injury Prevention*. Zatsiorsky V, ed. Oxford, UK: Blackwell Science, 2000, pp 349-362.

59. Kraemer W and Looney D. Underlying mechanisms and physiology of muscular power. *Strength and Cond J* 34: 13-19, 2012.

60. Kulig K, Andrews J, and Hay J. Human strength curves. *Exerc Sport Sci Rev* 12: 417-466, 1984.

61. Kuntz C, Masi M, and Lorenz D. Augmenting the bench press with elastic resistance: scientific and practical applications. *Strength and Cond J* 36: 96-102, 2014.

62. Lake J, Lauder M, Smith N, and Shorter K. A comparison of ballistic and nonballistic lower-body resistance exercise and the methods used to identify their positive lifting phases. *J Appl Biomech* 28: 431-437, 2012.

63. Lanka J. Shot putting, in: *Biomechanics in Sport: Performance Enhancement and Injury Prevention*. Zatsiorsky V, ed. Oxford, UK: Blackwell Science, 2000, pp 435-457.

64. Lyttle A, Wilson G, and Ostrowski K. Enhancing performance: maximal power versus combined weights and plyometric training. *J Strength Cond Res* 10, 1996.

65. MacKenzie S, Lavers R, and Wallace B. A biomechanical comparison of the vertical jump, power clean, and jump squat. *J Sport Sci* 1632: 1576-1585, 2014.

66. Maio Alves J, Rebelo A, Abrantes C, and Sampaio J. Short-term effects of complex and contrast training in soccer players' vertical jump, sprint, and agility abilities. *J Strength Cond Res* 24: 936-941, 2010.

67. Markovic G and Jaric S. Positive and negative loading and mechanical output in maximum vertical jumping. *Med Sci Sports Exerc* 39: 1757-1764, 2007.

68. Markovic G, Vuk S, and Jaric S. Effects of jump training with negative versus positive loading on jumping mechanics. *Int J Sports Med* 32: 365-372, 2011.

69. McBride J, Triplett-McBride N, Davie A, and Newton M. The effect of heavy- vs. light-load jump squats on the development of strength, power, and speed. *J Strength Cond Res* 16: 72-82, 2002.

70. McMaster D, Cronin J, and McGuigan M. Forms of variable resistance training. *J Strength Cond Res* 31: 50-64, 2009.

71. McMaster D, Cronin J, and McGuigan M. Quantification of rubber and chain-based resistance modes. *J Strength Cond Res* 24: 2056-2064, 2010.

72. Mero A and Komi P. Force-, EMG-, and elasticity-velocity relationships at submaximal, maximal and supramaximal running speeds in sprinters. *Eur J Appl Physiol Occup Physiol* 55: 553-561, 1986.

73. Miller D. Springboard and platform diving, in: *Biomechanics in Sport: Performance Enhancement and Injury Prevention*. Zatsiorsky V, ed. Oxford, UK: Blackwell Science, 2000, pp 326-348.

74. Neelly K, Terry J, and Morris M. A mechanical comparison of linear and double-looped hung supplemental heavy chain resistance to the back squat: a case study. *J Strength Cond Res* 24: 278-281, 2010.

75. Newton R and Kraemer W. Developing explosive muscular power: implications for a mixed methods training strategy. *Strength and Cond J* 16: 20-31, 1994.

76. Newton R, Kraemer W, and Hakkinen K. Effects of ballistic training on preseason preparation of elite volleyball players. *Med Sci Sports Exerc* 31: 323-330, 1999.

77. Newton R, Kraemer W, Hakkinen K, Humphries B, and Murphy A. Kinematics, kinetics, and muscle activation during explosive upper body movements. *J Appl Biomech* 12: 31-43, 1996.

78. Newton R, Murphy A, Humphries B, Wilson G, Kraemer W, and Hakkinen K. Influence of load and stretch shortening cycle on the kinematics, kinetics and muscle activation that occurs during explosive bench press throws. *Eur J Appl Physiol Occup Physiol* 75: 333-342, 1997.

79. Paasuke M, Ereline J, and Gapeyeva H. Twitch potentiation capacity of plantar-flexor muscles in endurance and power athletes. *Biol Sport* 15: 171-178, 1996.

80. Pereria M and Gomes P. Movement velocity in resistance training. *Sports Med* 33: 427-438, 2003.

81. Pipes T. Variable resistance versus constant resistance strength training in adult males. *Eur J Appl Physiol Occup Physiol* 39: 27-35, 1978.

82. Radcliffe J and Radcliffe J. Effects of different warm-up protocols on peak power output during a single response jump task. *Med Sci Sports Exerc* 38: S189, 1999.

83. Rajamohan G, Kanagasabai P, Krishnaswamy S, and Balakrishnan A. Effect of complex and contrast resistance and plyometric training on selected strength and power parameters. *J Exp Sciences* 1: 1-12, 2010.

84. Ramírez J, Núñez V, Lancho C, Poblador M, and Lancho J. Velocity based training of lower limb to improve absolute and relative power outputs in concentric phase of half-squat in soccer players. *J Strength Cond Res*, 29: 3084-3088, 2015.

85. Randell A, Cronin J, Keogh J, Gill N, and Pedersen M. Effect of instantaneous performance feedback during 6 weeks of velocity-based resistance training on sport-specific performance tests. *J Strength Cond Res* 25: 87-93, 2011.

86. Rhea M, Kenn J, and Dermody B. Alterations in speed of squat movement and the use of accommodated resistance among college athletes training for power. *J Strength Cond Res* 23: 2645-2650, 2009.

87. Robbins D. Postactivation potentiation and its practical applicability: a brief review. *J Strength Cond Res* 19: 453-458, 2005.

88. Sale D. Postactivation potentiation: role in human performance. *Exerc Sport Sci Rev* 30: 138-143, 2002.

89. Seitz L, Trajano G, Dal Maso F, Haff G, and Blazevich A. Postactivation potentiation during voluntary contractions after continued knee extensor task-specific practice. *Appl Physiol Nutr Metab* 40: 230-237, 2015.

90. Shea C, Kohl R, Guadagnoli M, and Shebilske W. After-contraction phenomenon: influences on performance and learning. *J Mot Behav* 23: 51-62, 1991.

91. Sheppard J, Dingley A, Janssen I, Spratford W, Chapman D, and Newton R. The effect of assisted jumping on vertical jump height in high-performance volleyball players. *J Sci Med Sport* 14: 85-89, 2011.

92. Soria-Gila M, Chirosa I, Bautista I, Chirosa L, and Salvador B. Effects of variable resistance training on maximal strength: a meta-analysis. *J Strength Cond Res*, 29: 3260-3270, 2015.

93. Sotiropoulos K, Smilios I, Douda H, Chritou M, and Tokmakidis S. Contrast loading: power output and rest interval effects on neuromuscular performance. *Int J Sports Physiol Perf* 9: 567-574, 2014.

94. Stone M, O'Bryant H, McCoy L, Coglianese R, Lehmkuhl M, and Schilling B. Power and maximal strength relationships during performance of dynamic and static weighted jumps. *J Strength Cond Res* 17: 140-147, 2003.

95. Stone M, Sanborn K, O'Bryant H, Hartman M, Stone M, Prouix C, Ward B, and Hruby J. Maximal strength-power-performance relationships in collegiate throwers. *J Strength Cond Res* 17: 739-745, 2003.

96. Stone M, Sands W, Pierce K, Ramsey M, and Haff G. Power and power potentiation among strength power athletes: preliminary study. *Int J Sports Physiol Perf* 3: 55-67, 2008.

97. Stone M, Stone M, and Sands W. *Principles and Practice of Resistance Training.* Champaign, IL: Human Kinetics, 2007.

98. Thomas K, French D, and Hayes P. The effects of two plyometric training techniques on muscular power and agility in youth soccer players. *J Strength Cond Res* 23: 332-335, 2009.

99. Tillin N and Bishop D. Factors modulating post-activation potentiation and its effect on performance of subsequent explosive activities. *Sports Med* 39: 147-166, 2009.

100. Turner A. Training for power: principles and practice. *Prof Strength Cond* 14: 20-32, 2009.

101. Verkhoshansky Y and Tatyan V. Speed-strength preparation for future champions. *Logkaya Atletika* 2: 2-13, 1973.

102. Verkhoshansky Y and Verkhoshansky N. *Special strength training manual for coaches.* Verkhoshansky.com, 2011.

103. Wallace B, Winchester J, and McGuigan M. Effects of elastic bands on force and power characteristics during the back squat exercise. *J Strength Cond Res* 20: 268-272, 2006.

104. Wilson G, Murphy A, and Walshe A. Performance benefits from weight and plyometric training: effects of initial strength level. *Coaching Sport Sci J* 2: 3-8, 1997.

105. Wilson G, Newton R, Murphy A, and Humphries B. The optimal training load for the development of dynamic athletic performance. *Med Sci Sports Exerc* 23: 1279-1286, 1993.

106. Wilson J and Kritz M. Practical guidelines and considerations for the use of elastic bands in strength and conditioning. *Strength and Cond J* 36: 1-9, 2014.

107. Young W, Jenner A, and Griffiths K. Acute enhancement of power performance from heavy load squats. *J Strength Cond Res* 12: 82-84, 1998.

108. Zatsiorsky V. Studies of motion and motor abilities of sportsmen, in: *Biomechanics IV.* Nelson R, Morehouse C, eds. Baltimore: University Park Press, 1974, pp 273-275.

109. Zatsiorsky V and Kraemer W. *Science and Practice of Strength Training.* Champaign, IL: Human Kinetics, 1995.

110. Zepeda P and Gonzalez J. Complex training: three weeks pre-season conditioning in Division I female basketball players. *J Strength Cond Res* 14: 372, 2000.

Chapter 9

1. Argus CK, Gill ND, Keogh JW, McGuigan MR, and Hopkins WG. Effects of two contrast training programs on jump performance in rugby union players during a competition phase. *Int J Sports Physiol Perform* 7: 68-75, 2012.

2. Bradbury JC and Forman SL. The impact of pitch counts and days of rest on performance among major-league baseball pitchers. *J Strength Cond Res* 26: 1181-1187, 2012.

3. Kilduff LP, Finn CV, Baker JS, Cook CJ, and West DJ. Preconditioning strategies to enhance physical performance on the day of competition. *Int J Sports Physiol Perform* 8: 677-681, 2013.

4. Newton RU, Rogers RA, Volek JS, Hakkinen K, and Kraemer WJ. Four weeks of optimal load ballistic resistance training at the end of season attenuates declining jump performance of women volleyball players. *J Strength Cond Res* 20: 955-961, 2006.

Chapter 10

1. Aagaard P and Andersen JL. Effects of strength training on endurance capacity in top-level endurance athletes. *Scand J Med Sci Sports* 20 Suppl 2: 39-47, 2010.

2. Beattie K, Kenny IC, Lyons M, and Carson BP. The effect of strength training on performance in endurance athletes. *Sports Med* 44: 845-865, 2014.

3. Bullock N, Martin DT, Ross A, Rosemond D, Holland T, and Marino FE. Characteristics of the start in women's World Cup skeleton. *Sports Biomech* 7: 351-360, 2008.

4. Kilduff LP, Finn CV, Baker JS, Cook CJ, and West DJ. Preconditioning strategies to enhance physical performance on the day of competition. *Int J Sports Physiol Perform* 8: 677-681, 2013.

5. Lawton TW, Cronin JB, and McGuigan MR. Strength testing and training of rowers: a review. *Sports Med* 41: 413-432, 2011.

6. Parchmann CJ and McBride JM. Relationship between functional movement screen and athletic performance. *J Strength Cond Res* 25: 3378-3384, 2011.

7. Ronnestad BR, Kojedal O, Losnegard T, Kvamme B, and Raastad T. Effect of heavy strength training on muscle thickness, strength, jump performance, and endurance performance in well-trained Nordic Combined athletes. *Eur J Appl Physiol Occup Physiol* 112: 2341-2352, 2012.

Index

Note: Page references followed by an italicized *f* or *t* indicate information contained in figures or tables, respectively.

About the NSCA

The National Strength and Conditioning Association (NSCA) is the world's leading organization in the field of sport conditioning. Drawing on the resources and expertise of the most recognized professionals in strength training and conditioning, sport science, performance research, education, and sports medicine, the NSCA is the world's trusted source of knowledge and training guidelines for coaches and athletes. The NSCA provides the crucial link between the lab and the field.

About the Editor

Mike R. McGuigan, PhD, CSCS, is a professor of strength and conditioning at Auckland University of Technology (AUT) in New Zealand. From 2009 through 2012, he was a sport scientist with High Performance Sport New Zealand, where he worked with many elite athletes. He has worked in a variety of academic roles at universities in Australia and in the United States.

Dr. McGuigan is an associate editor for the *Journal of Australian Strength and Conditioning, Journal of Strength and Conditioning Research*, and *International Journal of Sports Physiology and Performance*. He was the research and innovation coordinator for the New Zealand Silver

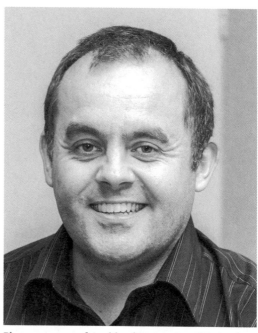

Photo courtesy of Auckland University of Technology

Ferns netball team from 2009 to 2015. His research interests are areas of strength and power development and monitoring athletes.

Dr. McGuigan was the recipient of the NSCA's William J. Kraemer Outstanding Sport Scientist of the Year award in 2016, the *Journal of Strength and Conditioning Research* Editorial Excellence Award in 2010, and the National Strength and Conditioning Association Outstanding Young Investigator Award in 2007. He lives in Auckland, New Zealand.

About the Contributors

Duncan N. French, PhD, CSCS,*D, is the Vice President of Performance at the UFC Performance Institute. Prior to this, Dr. French was the Director of Performance Sciences at Notre Dame University, where he also serves as the Director of Olympic Sport Strength and Conditioning. Previously, Dr. French was a Technical Lead for Strength and Conditioning at the English Institute of Sport, and he has acted as the National Lead for Strength and Conditioning to both Great Britain Taekwondo and Great Britain Basketball's Olympic programs. He has coached Olympic, World Championship, and Commonwealth Games medalists from a vari-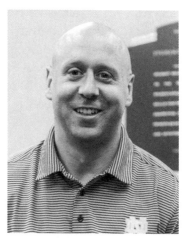ety of sporting disciplines, and he was the Head of Strength and Conditioning at Newcastle United Football Club. He holds a PhD in Exercise Physiology from the University of Connecticut, and has authored or co-authored over 55 peer-reviewed scientific manuscripts. Dr. French is a former Chairman of the United Kingdom Strength and Conditioning Association.

G. Gregory Haff, PhD, CSCS,*D, FNSCA, is an associate professor and course coordinator in the Masters of Exercise Science (Strength and Conditioning) at Edith Cowan University. He is President of the National Strength and Conditioning Association and serves as a Sport Scientist on the Australian Weightlifting High Performance Program Panel. Dr. Haff is an Australian Strength and Conditioning Association Level 2 Strength Coach. In 2014, he was named the United Kingdom Strength and Conditioning Association: Strength and Conditioning Coach of the Year for Education and Research. Additionally, in 2011, he was awarded the NSCA's William J. Kraemer Sport Scientist of the Year 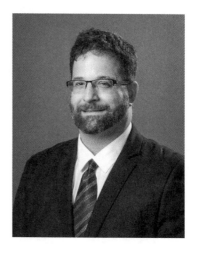Award. Dr. Haff is a Level 3 Australian Weightlifting Association Coach and a NSCA Certified Strength and Conditioning Specialist with Distinction.

Disa L. Hatfield, PhD, CSCS,*D, is currently an associate professor at the University of Rhode Island in the Department of Kinesiology. Dr. Hatfield is certified by the NSCA as a Strength and Conditioning Specialist and has served on the NSCA's Education, Research, and Nominating committees. She is a senior Associate Editor for the *Journal of Strength and Conditioning*. Dr. Hatfield has over 40 published research articles in the areas of strength and power, hormonal responses to resistance exercise, and children and exercise. She is also a 3-time U.S.A.P.L. National Champion Powerlifter, I.O.C. World Games athlete, and 2-time American Bench Press record holder.

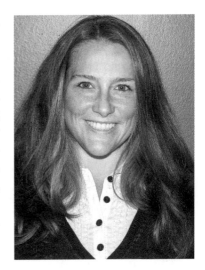

Rhodri S. Lloyd, PhD, CSCS,*D, is a Senior Lecturer in Strength and Conditioning and Chair of the Youth Physical Development Centre at Cardiff Metropolitan University. He also holds research associate and fellowship positions with Auckland University of Technology and Waikato Institute of Technology. His research interests include the impact of growth and maturation on long-term athletic development and the neuromuscular mechanisms underpinning resistance training adaptations in youth. He is an associate editor for

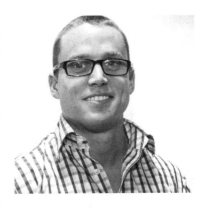

the *Journal of Strength and Conditioning Research* and the *Strength and Conditioning Journal*. In 2016, he received the Strength and Conditioning Coach of the Year award for Research and Education by the United Kingdom Strength and Conditioning Association (UKSCA). Previously, he served as a Board Director for the UKSCA. Currently, he is Chair of the National Strength and Conditioning Association's (NSCA) Youth Training Special Interest Group.

Jeffrey M. McBride, PhD, CSCS, is a professor in Exercise Science at Appalachian State University in the Department of Health and Exercise Science. He is also the Director of the Neuromuscular and Biomechanics Laboratory. Dr. McBride was a post-doctoral fellow at the University of Jyvaskyla in Finland and he received his PhD in Human Movement from Southern Cross University in Australia. He completed his Master's Degree in Exercise Physiology at Penn State and his Bachelor's Degree in Exercise Science from West Virginia University. He was awarded the Outstanding Young Investigator Award in 2006 from the National Strength and Conditioning Association. He is also a fellow of this same organization. He has published 86 manuscripts in scientific journals and has 128 conference abstract presentations.

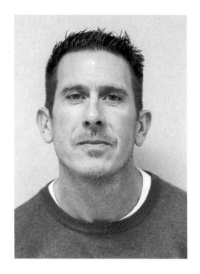

Sophia Nimphius, PhD, CSCS,*D, is an associate professor in the School of Medical and Health Sciences at Edith Cowan University. She is the sport science manager at the Hurley Surfing Australia High Performance Centre and manages High Performance Services for Softball Western Australia. Dr. Nimphius is a National Strength and Conditioning Association (NSCA) certified strength and conditioning specialist, an Australian Strength and Conditioning Association (ASCA) Pro-Scheme Accredited Coach – Elite, and a Level 2 Accredited Sports Scientist with Exercise and Sports Science Australia (ESSA).

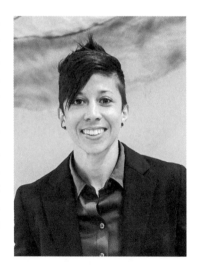

Jeremy M. Sheppard, PhD, CSCS, has been a strength and conditioning coach since 1994. At present, he is the Director of Performance Services at the Canadian Sport Institute in the Pacific, and the Sport Science and Medicine Lead for Canada Snowboard. Previously, he worked with or led performance programs with Surfing Australia, Queensland Academy of Sport, Australian Institute of Sport, Australian Volleyball Federation, and Canadian Sport Centre. He has also consulted with professional sports leagues, including the NFL, the NRL, and the AFL.

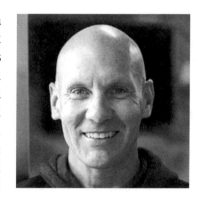

Adam Storey, PhD, is a research fellow at AUT University's Sports Performance Research Institute (New Zealand) where he supervises post-graduate research in the areas of strength and conditioning and exercise physiology. From 2008 – 2016, he coached and managed various New Zealand weightlifting teams at key pinnacle events including the 2012 and 2016 Olympic Games and the 2010 and 2014 Commonwealth Games. During this time, Dr. Storey coached weightlifters to Commonwealth Games medals and his athletes broke over 250 New Zealand records in competition. His specialist background in the area of strength and power conditioning lead to his role with High Per-

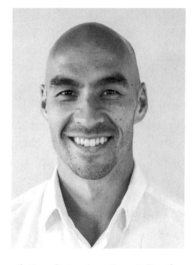

formance Sport New Zealand as the Lead Strength and Conditioning Specialist for Athletics New Zealand. Dr. Storey has a keen passion for rugby. He is currently the Sports Science Manager and Assistant Trainer for the Blues Super Rugby franchise.

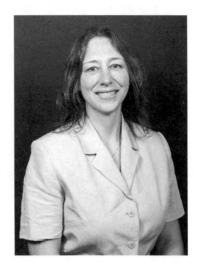

N. Travis Triplett, PhD, CSCS,*D, FNSCA, is a professor and Director of the Strength and Conditioning Concentrations for the Bachelor and Master of Science degrees in Exercise Science at Appalachian State University. Her past experience includes a being director of the Strength Centers at the University of Wisconsin-La Crosse, a research assistantship in Sports Physiology at the US Olympic Training Center in Colorado Springs, and a postdoctoral research fellowship at Southern Cross University in Australia. She also has completed international research at the University of Jyvaskyla in Finland and at the University of Valencia in Spain. Dr. Triplett is currently a senior associate editor for the *Journal of Strength and Conditioning Research*. She was a past assistant editor-in-chief for the *Strength and Conditioning Journal*. She received the 2010 William J. Kraemer Outstanding Sport Scientist Award, the 2000 Terry J. Housh Outstanding Young Investigator award, and the 2016 JSCR Editorial Excellence Award. She also served on two panels for NASA, including one for developing resistance exercise countermeasures to micro-gravity environments for the International Space Station. Dr. Triplett holds certification from USA Weightlifting in addition to her NSCA certification.

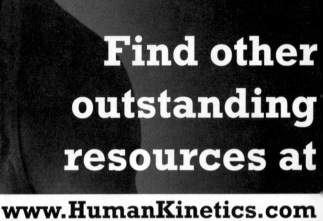